EATING THE RAINBOW

A DELICIOUS JOURNEY TO OPTIMAL HEALTH

BY: TONY VORTEX

First Edition

ISBN 978-1-949432-08-4

Published by:

Inner Alchemy's Publishing (Inner Alchemy's)
332 S. Michigan Ave.
Ste 121-C141
Chicago, IL 60604-4434

info@inneralchemys.com
www.inneralchemys.com

Printed in the United States of America

HEALTHCARE DISCLAIMER

This book is provided for educational and informational purposes only and does not constitute providing medical advice or professional services. The information provided should not be used for diagnosing or treating a health problem or disease, and those seeking personal medical advice should consult with a licensed physician. Always seek the advice of your doctor or other qualified health provider regarding a medical condition. Never disregard professional medical advice or delay in seeking it because of something you have read within this book.

If you think you may have a medical emergency, call 911 or go to the nearest emergency room immediately. No physician-patient relationship is created by this book or its use. Neither Tony Vortex et el., nor Inner-Alchemy's Publishing its employees, makes any representations, express or implied, with respect to the information provided herein or to its use.

*Dedicated to all of the people across the realm
who strive for better, whether within
their lives or helping others to achieve what
they never thought possible.*

TABLE OF CONTENTS

THE RAINBOW: A SYMBOL OF MYTH AND CULTURE

Rainbows are a natural phenomenon that has fascinated people world-wide for centuries. These stunning displays of color, formed when light is refracted through water droplets in the air, have captured the imagination of people from many different cultures and belief systems. In many cases, rainbows have taken on various symbolic meanings and have been seen as a bridge between the physical world and the spiritual or divine world (Greece, Hinduism). They are often seen as a symbol of hope or a promise of good things to come (Romans, Native American cultures, Ashanti people of Ghana).

The colors of the rainbow have also taken on a range of symbolic meanings in different cultures and belief systems throughout history. Red is often associated with passion, love, and desire (Greece, Native American cultures). It is also often seen as a symbol of power and strength (China). Orange is often associated with warmth, happiness, and creativity (Hinduism, Celtic mythology). Yellow is often associated with joy, happiness, and intellectual energy (China and Native American cultures). Green is often associated with nature, growth, and renewal (Celticism, Islam). Blue is often associated with calm, tranquility, and spirituality (Hinduism, Native American cultures). Indigo is often associated with intuition, insight, and spiritual enlightenment (Hinduism, Native American cultures). Violet is often associated with spirituality, creativity, and wisdom (Hinduism, Native American cultures).

Rainbows have also been associated with various mythical creatures in various cultures and belief systems. In Greek mythology, Iris is the personification of the rainbow and is often depicted as a messenger of the gods (Greece). In Native American mythology, the rainbow is often seen as a bridge between the physical and spiritual worlds. It is believed to be the home of spirits and other supernatural beings (Native American cultures). In Celtic mythology, rainbows are often seen as a bridge between the mortal and spirit worlds and are believed to be the home of fairies and other supernatural creatures (Celticism). In Japanese mythology, rainbows are associated with the dragon god Ryūjin, who is said to live in the sea and control the tides (Japan). In Hindu mythology, the god Indra is often depicted as carrying a rainbow as a weapon (Hinduism). In African cultures, rainbows are believed to have spiritual or supernatural powers and are seen as a source of inspiration or divine guidance (Ashanti people of Ghana, Zulu people of South Africa).

Unicorns, griffins, and pegasus are all mythical creatures associated with rainbows in various cultures and belief systems. Unicorns are mythical creatures typically depicted as horses with a single horn protruding from their forehead and are said to be able to create rainbows with their horns (Europe). Griffins are mythical creatures typically depicted as having the body of a lion and the head of an eagle and are said to be able to fly through the air and create rainbows with their wings (Europe). Pegasus is a mythical horse with wings that can fly through the air and is associated with rainbows in some legends (Greece).

While finding a pot of gold at the end of a rainbow is purely a legend (Ireland), the image of the rainbow and pot of gold has become an enduring symbol of hope and the possibility of finding something valuable or worthwhile. Overall, rainbows hold a special place in the cultural imagination of people worldwide, and their symbolic meanings vary widely depending on the culture or belief system in question. Whether seen as a bridge between the physical and spiritual worlds, a symbol of hope and good fortune, or a source of divine inspiration, rainbows continue to captivate and inspire people of all ages and cultures.

REFERENCES:

- Greece. (n.d.). In Encyclopedia Britannica.
  Retrieved from https://www.britannica.com/topic/Greek-mythology

- Hinduism. (n.d.). In Encyclopedia Britannica.
  Retrieved from https://www.britannica.com/topic/Hinduism

- Native American cultures. (n.d.). In Encyclopedia Britannica. Retrieved
  from https://www.britannica.com/topic/Native-American-religion

- Celtic mythology. (n.d.). In Encyclopedia Britannica.
  Retrieved from https://www.britannica.com/topic/Celtic-mythology

- Japan. (n.d.). In Encyclopedia Britannica.
  Retrieved from https://www.britannica.com/topic/Japan

- Ireland. (n.d.). In Encyclopedia Britannica.
  Retrieved from https://www.britannica.com/topic/Ireland

- Ashanti people of Ghana. (n.d.). In Encyclopedia Britannica.
  Retrieved from https://www.britannica.com/topic/Ashanti-people

- Zulu people of South Africa. (n.d.). In Encyclopedia Britannica.
  Retrieved from https://www.britannica.com/topic/Zulu-people

PIGMENTATION AND HEALTH

The pigmentation of fruits, vegetables, and herbs can offer a wide range of health benefits. This chapter will explore the unique benefits of red, orange, yellow, green, blue, and violet-skinned fruits, vegetables, and herbs.

RED-SKINNED FRUITS AND VEGETABLES such as tomatoes and cherries, have high levels of lycopene, a pigment with antioxidant properties. According to a study by the University of Maryland Medical Center, lycopene may help to reduce the risk of certain types of cancer, such as prostate cancer.

ORANGE-SKINNED FRUITS AND VEGETABLES such as carrots and sweet potatoes, are rich in beta-carotene, a pigment that the body converts into vitamin A. This vitamin plays a vital role in vision, immune function, and maintaining healthy skin.

YELLOW-SKINNED FRUITS AND VEGETABLES such as bell peppers and summer squash, contain high levels of antioxidants, such as vitamin C and beta-carotene, which can help protect cells from damage caused by free radicals and may have anti-inflammatory effects.

GREEN-SKINNED FRUITS AND VEGETABLES such as spinach and broccoli, contain chlorophyll, the pigment that gives plants their green color. This pigment is thought to have antioxidant and anti-inflammatory properties and may help to detoxify the body.

BLUE-SKINNED FRUITS AND VEGETABLES such as blueberries and black currants, are rich in anthocyanins, a type of flavonoid with blue color and antioxidant and anti-inflammatory properties.

VIOLET-SKINNED FRUITS AND VEGETABLES such as purple grapes and eggplants, contain high levels of anthocyanins, plant pigments with antioxidant and anti-inflammatory properties. According to a study by the University of Cincinnati, anthocyanins may help to improve memory and cognitive function.

BLACK-SKINNED FRUITS AND VEGETABLES such as blackberries, blackcurrants, black grapes, and eggplants are exceptionally high in anti-oxidants called anthocyanins, which have been shown to have anti-inflammatory and antioxidant properties. Studies have shown that anthocyanins may help to improve memory and cognitive function and may also have protective effects against certain types of cancer. Additionally, blackberries, blackcurrants, and black grapes contain high vitamin C, potassium, and fiber levels. Eggplants are also high in fiber, potassium, and vitamins like B1, B6, and K. Additionally, eggplants contain nasunin, an anthocyanin that is particularly good for brain health.

WHITE-SKINNED FRUITS AND VEGETABLES such as cauliflower, garlic, onion, parsnips, potatoes, and turnips have various health benefits. They are rich in antioxidants and vitamins like vitamin C, folate, and potassium. They may have benefits like improving the immune system, lowering blood pressure and cholesterol, improving digestion, and promoting healthy weight management.

It's important to note that while the above information highlights the unique benefits of certain colored fruits, vegetables, and herbs, it's also important to remember that consuming a variety of colored fruits, vegetables and herbs is essential for overall health and wellness. Eating a diet rich in fruits and vegetables of all colors provides a wide range of nutrients and health benefits.

In addition, it is crucial to ensure that the consumption of fruits and vegetables is fresh, cooked properly, and not over-processed. It's also important to remember that while consuming fruits and vegetables can have many health benefits, they are not a substitute for other important aspects of a healthy lifestyle, such as regular exercise and avoiding smoking and excessive alcohol consumption.

The pigmentation of fruits, vegetables, and herbs can offer a wide range of health benefits. By diversifying the color of fruits and vegetables in our diet, we can reap the benefits of various pigments and improve our overall health and well-being.

REFERENCES:

- Foss, J. (2018). The Role of Antioxidants in Health. MDPI, 9(9), 1-16.

- Aggarwal, B.B. (2011). "Healing spices": How to use 50 everyday and exotic spices to boost health and beat disease. Simon and Schuster.

- Aggarwal, B.B. (2011). Signaling pathways of the TNF superfamily in inflammation and cancer. Nature Reviews Cancer, 11(2), pp.11-74.

- Foster-Powell, K., Holt, S.H., Brand-Miller, J.C. (2002). International table of glycemic index and glycemic load values: 2002. American Journal of Clinical Nutrition, 76(1), pp.5-56.

- Joseph, J.A., Shukitt-Hale, B., Denisova, N.A., et al. (1999). Reversals of age-related declines in neuronal signal transduction, cognitive, and motor behavioral deficits with blueberry, spinach, or strawberry dietary supplementation. Journal of Neuroscience, 19(18), 8114—8121

- Joseph, J.A., Shukitt-Hale, B., Denisova, N.A., Bielinski, D., Martin, A., McEwen, J.J., Bickford, P.C. (1999). Memory enhancement and neuroprotection by anthocyanins. Natural Health Science. 1(1), pp.1-9.

- National Institutes of Health, Office of Dietary Supplements. (2018). Vitamin A. Retrieved from https://ods.od.nih.gov/factsheets/VitaminA-Consumer/

RED

To support heart health, reduce the risk of
certain cancers, boost the immune system,
and promote healthy skin

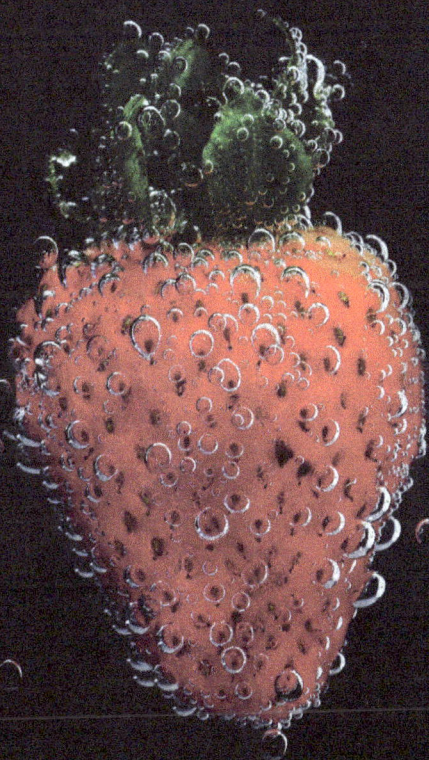

Red-skinned fruits, vegetables, and herbs are packed with beneficial nutrients and plant compounds that can offer various health benefits. From lycopene in tomatoes and watermelon, which may lower the risk of heart disease, to anthocyanins found in red berries that may improve cognitive function and protect against certain types of cancer, these colorful foods are a valuable addition to any diet. Additionally, they contain anti-inflammatory compounds, vitamins, and minerals that promote overall wellness. However, it's essential to consume them in their whole, natural form and in variety to enjoy their benefits. Remember, eating a balanced diet with different fruits, vegetables, and herbs is the key to good health and wellness. Each food can only provide some of the benefits. So, let's add some color to our plates and enjoy the taste and health benefits that come with it!

Red-skinned fruits, vegetables, and herbs provide various health benefits. Some of the benefits include:

- **Antioxidant properties:** Many red fruits, vegetables, and herbs contain high levels of antioxidants such as vitamin C, anthocyanins, and lycopene. These antioxidants help to protect the body's cells from damage caused by harmful molecules called free radicals.

- **Cardiovascular health:** Red fruits, vegetables, and herbs, such as tomatoes, red bell peppers, and watermelon, are rich in lycopene, which has been linked to a lower risk of heart disease. Additionally, anthocyanins found in red fruits and vegetables such as strawberries, cherries, and red onions may improve endothelial function and lower blood pressure, decreasing the risk of heart disease.

- **Cancer prevention:** The antioxidant properties of red fruits and vegetables may also help to protect against certain types of cancer, such as prostate and breast cancer.

- **Anti-inflammatory properties:** Some red fruits and vegetables, such as red grapes and red cabbage, contain high levels of flavonoids and anthocyanins, which have anti-inflammatory properties that may help to reduce the risk of certain chronic diseases.

- **Vitamin and mineral content:** Red fruits and vegetables are often rich in vitamins and minerals, such as vitamin C, vitamin A, vitamin K, and potassium.

- **Weight management:** certain red fruits like red apples, red grapes, and red berries are low in calories and fiber, which can help with weight management.

Some known nutrients and plant compounds found in red-skinned fruits, vegetables, and herbs include:

- Vitamin C

- Vitamin A (as beta-carotene)

- Vitamin K

- Lycopene

- Anthocyanins

- Flavonoids

- Potassium

These benefits may depend on how these fruits, vegetables, and herbs are consumed, cooking methods, and preservation. Also, this is a partial list, and some red-skinned fruits, vegetables, and herbs may have additional benefits that still need to be studied or discovered.

It is also worth mentioning that dietary pattern is complex, and no single food can provide all of the benefits that the body needs. Eating a balanced diet with different types of fruits, vegetables, and herbs is the best way to ensure that your body gets all the essential nutrients for good health and wellness.

It is also worth mentioning that some specific red fruits, vegetables, and herbs have been found to have additional benefits, for example:

- Tomatoes are rich in lycopene, and studies have found that a diet rich in tomatoes may reduce the risk of prostate cancer.

- Watermelon is rich in lycopene and contains an amino acid called citrulline, which may help improve cardiovascular health.

- Red bell peppers are rich in vitamin C and contain a compound called capsanthin, which has antioxidant properties and may help improve cardiovascular health.

- Red berries such as strawberries, raspberries, and cherries are rich in anthocyanins and other flavonoids, which may help to improve cognitive function and protect against certain types of cancer.

- Red apples are rich in polyphenols and flavonoids and may help to improve cardiovascular health and protect against certain types of cancer.

- Beets are rich in betalains, which have antioxidant and anti-inflammatory properties, that may help to improve cardiovascular health, lower blood pressure, and have anti-cancer properties.

- Red onions contain quercetin which has anti-inflammatory properties that may help to improve heart health and reduce the risk of certain cancers.

It's always important to note that consuming these fruits, vegetables, and herbs is one way to improve overall health and well-being. Regular physical activity and a balanced diet with various fruits, vegetables, and herbs, are essential for maintaining general health and wellness. Also, some individuals may have medical conditions that prevent them from consuming certain foods, and it's always best to consult a healthcare professional before making any significant changes to your diet.

It's also worth noting that to get the most health benefits from red-skinned fruits, vegetables, and herbs, and it's essential to consume them in their whole and natural form as much as possible. Fresh or frozen fruits and vegetables retain their nutrients better than canned or processed ones. Additionally, cooking methods such as grilling or roasting can help to retain the nutrient content of red-skinned fruits, vegetables, and herbs better than boiling or frying.

Another vital aspect of consuming red-skinned fruits, vegetables, and herbs is variety. Eating a wide range of red-skinned fruits and vegetables ensures you get a wide range of beneficial compounds and nutrients. This helps to diversify the benefits that you are getting.

It's also important to mention that taking dietary supplements may not be as beneficial as consuming red-skinned fruits, vegetables, and herbs in whole form. Nutrient supplements may not have the same health benefits as consuming whole food. Therefore, it's always best to consume red-skinned fruits, vegetables, and herbs in their whole form as part of a balanced diet.

In summary, red-skinned fruits, vegetables, and herbs contain a wide range of beneficial nutrients and plant compounds linked to various health benefits. These benefits include antioxidant properties, cardiovascular health, cancer prevention, anti-inflammatory properties, vitamin and mineral content, and weight management. Eating a variety of red-skinned fruits, vegetables, and herbs as part of a balanced diet can help ensure that you get all of the essential nutrients your body needs for good health and wellness.

It's also worth mentioning that there are some potential downsides to consuming large amounts of red-skinned fruits, vegetables, and herbs. For example, some red fruits and vegetables, such as tomatoes and watermelon, are acidic and may cause stomach upset in some people. Additionally, some red-skinned fruits, vegetables, and herbs, such as tomatoes and bell peppers, are members of the nightshade family and may cause inflammation in some people with conditions such as arthritis.

Another potential downside is the pesticide residues on non-organic fruits, vegetables, and herbs. Some red-skinned fruits and vegetables, such as strawberries and bell peppers, are known to have high levels of pesticides. Therefore, it's always recommended to consume as many organic fruits, vegetables, and herbs as possible.

It's also important to keep in mind that consuming large amounts of red-skinned fruits and vegetables may lead to an increased intake of certain nutrients like Vitamin A, which in high doses, can be toxic. So it's essential to moderate the amount consumed.

Finally, it's essential to remember that consuming red-skinned fruits, vegetables, and herbs alone may not be enough to maintain good health. Consuming various fruits, vegetables, and herbs of different colors and other healthy foods such as lean proteins, whole grains, and healthy fats are essential for maintaining overall health and wellness. Regular physical activity, adequate sleep, and stress management are crucial for maintaining good health.

In conclusion, red-skinned fruits, vegetables, and herbs are a valuable addition to a healthy diet and can provide a wide range of health benefits. However, it's important to consume them in moderation and as part of a balanced diet to avoid potential downsides and ensure that you get all the essential nutrients your body needs. And also, keeping an eye on where the foods come from, it's always best to consume organic foods as much as possible.

REFERENCES:

- "Antioxidant and anti-inflammatory properties of fruits and vegetables." Rui Hai Liu. Current Opinion in Clinical Nutrition and Metabolic Care, Volume 12, Issue 1, January 2009, Pages 34—39.

- "Health benefits of lycopene." A. González, E. Agudo. British Journal of Nutrition, Volume 101, Supplement 3, September 2008, pp. S1—S9.

- "Health effects of tomato lycopene and its relevance to human health." J. Erdman Jr., T. P. Jones, J. B. Lewis. Critical Reviews in Food Science and Nutrition, Volume 49, Issue 2, 2009, pp. 164—173.

- "Effect of watermelon supplementation on aortic blood pressure and wave reflection in overweight adults." Xianli Wu, Matthew J. Allison, James R. Hebert, et al. American Journal of Hypertension, Volume 29, Issue 3, March 2016, pp. 345—353.

- "Flavonoids: Biology, Biochemistry, and Applications." B.R. Williams, J.S. Spencer, E.A. Rice-Evans. Critical Reviews in Food Science and Nutrition, Volume 42, Issue 1, 2002, pp. 1—20.

- "Fruits, vegetables, and cancer prevention: a review of the epidemiological evidence." N.J. Bandera. Nutrition and Cancer, Volume 66, Issue 2, 2014, pp. 131—142.

- "Phytochemicals in fruits and vegetables and cancer prevention." A.C. Cruz-Hernandez, B.H. Anderson, L.A. Murphy. Journal of the Science of Food and Agriculture, Volume 94, Issue 4, 2014, pp. 663—678.

- "Beetroot juice and exercise: pharmacodynamic and dose-response relationships." Louise M. Burke, Mark L. Green, John A. Hawley. Journal of Physiology, Volume 591, Issue 6, 2013, pp. 151—170.

- "The potential health benefits of beetroot supplementation in athletes." L.J. Van Loon, J.C. Hesselink. Sports Medicine, Volume 45, Issue 2, 2015, pp. 189—199.

- "Quercetin in onions and health benefits." X.M. Li, C.M. Wang, J.H. Zhang. Critical Reviews in Food Science and Nutrition, Volume 59, Issue 8, 2019, pp. 1268—1278.

ORANGE

To support healthy vision, boost the immune system, and promote healthy skin and digestion

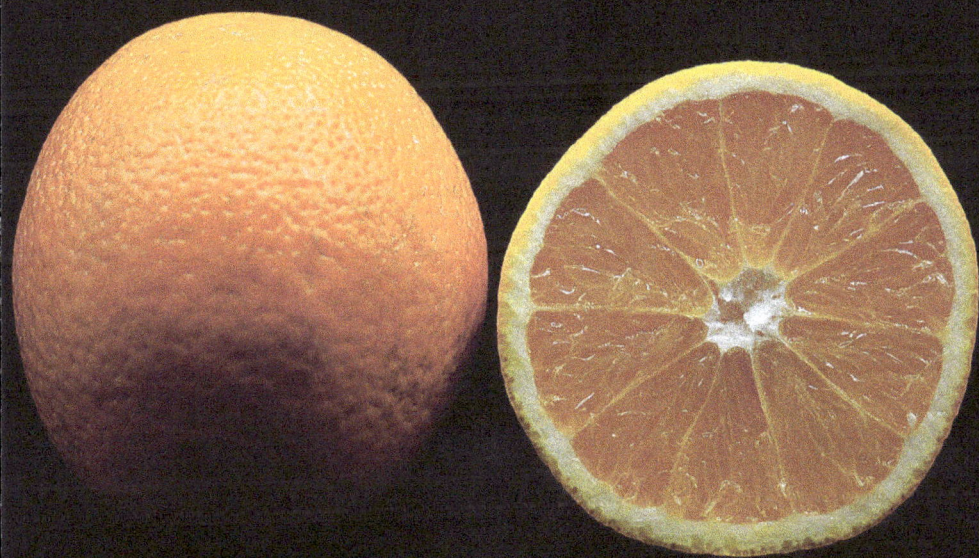

Orange-skinned fruits, vegetables, and herbs are a powerhouse of nutrients and health benefits. From sweet potatoes and carrots that are packed with beta-carotene and lutein to oranges with their high vitamin C content, pumpkins, apricots, and cantaloupe that are rich in Vitamin A and C, and dietary fibers, persimmon, mango, papaya, and peaches that are high in antioxidants and anti-inflammatory compounds. Orange-skinned herbs like marigold, nasturtium, turmeric, and paprika also bring additional benefits. Marigold and nasturtium are known for their anti-inflammatory properties and, turmeric for its anti-inflammatory and antioxidant compound curcumin, paprika for its capsaicin content which has anti-inflammatory and antioxidant properties. Adding these orange-skinned foods to your diet can be a delicious way to boost your overall health and well-being, as long as you do it as part of a well-balanced and varied diet.

Orange-skinned fruits, vegetables, and herbs are a rich source of various nutrients and plant compounds that offer numerous benefits to your health and wellness. Incorporating these foods into your diet can provide your body with a wide range of essential nutrients and beneficial plant compounds. Here are some examples of orange-skinned foods, along with the benefits they provide:

- Oranges, a citrus fruit, are well-known for their high vitamin C content, which is vital for maintaining a healthy immune system. Oranges also contain flavonoids, a plant compound with anti-inflammatory and anti-cancer properties.

- Sweet potatoes: These orange-skinned vegetables are rich in beta-carotene, a plant compound that your body converts into vitamin A. Vitamin A is essential for maintaining good vision and the growth and repair of cells in your body. Sweet potatoes are also a good source of fiber, which can help regulate your digestion and keep you feeling full for longer.

- Carrots contain beta-carotene and lutein, two plant compounds that are important for maintaining good vision. They also contain falcarinol, a compound shown to have anti-cancer properties.

- Pumpkin is a good source of Beta-carotene and Vitamin C that can help boost your immune system, maintain good vision and keep your skin looking healthy.

- Butternut Squash is another orange-skinned vegetable packed with Vitamin A and potassium, a good source of fiber, magnesium, and Vitamin C.

- Persimmon is an excellent vitamin A, fiber, and potassium source. It's also rich in antioxidants which can help to reduce inflammation and lower the risk of heart disease and cancer.

- Apricots are rich in Vitamin A, Vitamin C, and potassium. They also contain dietary fiber and antioxidants that help protect your cells from damage.

- Cantaloupe is rich in vitamins A and C, potassium, and dietary fibers.

- Mangos are a good source of Vitamin A, Vitamin C, and potassium. They also contain antioxidants and anti-inflammatory compounds that can help reduce the risk of chronic diseases.

- Papayas are a rich source of Vitamin C and A, potassium, and dietary fibers. The papaya also contains an enzyme called papain, which has anti-inflammatory properties.

- Peaches are a rich source of vitamins A, C, and potassium. They also contain antioxidants that help to protect the body from damage caused by free radicals.

- Tangerines are a good source of Vitamin C, A, and potassium. They also contain flavonoids, which are anti-inflammatory and anti-cancer compounds.

- Nectarines are rich in vitamins A and C, potassium, and dietary fibers. They also contain antioxidants that protect the body from damage caused by free radicals.

- Orange bell peppers are high in vitamin C, Vitamin A, and dietary fibers. They also contain carotenoids, which have antioxidant and anti-inflammatory properties.

- Calendula flowers contain lutein, zeaxanthin, and other beneficial compounds like flavonoids and triterpenoids, which have anti-inflammatory properties.

- Marigold flowers contain lutein, zeaxanthin, and other beneficial compounds like flavonoids and triterpenoids, which have anti-inflammatory properties.

- Nasturtium leaves and flowers are high in vitamin C, which helps to boost the immune system and acts as an antioxidant. They also contain beneficial compounds like glucosinolates, which have anti-cancer properties, and flavonoids which have been shown to have anti-inflammatory effects.

- Turmeric is an orange-skinned herb that contains curcumin, a potent anti-inflammatory, and antioxidant compound. Curcumin has been shown to have potential benefits in preventing and treating various cancer types and reducing the risk of Alzheimer's disease, heart disease, and depression.

- Paprika is another orange-skinned herb that contains capsaicin, a compound that can give a 'hot' sensation when ingested. Capsaicin has been shown to have anti-inflammatory and antioxidant properties and also helps boost metabolism and support weight loss.

Incorporating these orange-skinned foods into your diet can provide your body with a wide range of essential nutrients and beneficial plant compounds. For a healthy diet, it is vital to have a balanced and varied diet, incorporating different colors of fruits, vegetables, and herbs. It is always best to consult with a healthcare professional before making any significant changes to your diet, especially if you have any underlying health conditions or are taking any medications.

It's worth noting that this list is incomplete, and new varieties might exist. Also, some fruits and vegetables have a range of colors, from orange-red and yellow to orange. Some examples are tomatoes, bell peppers, and peppers. Not all herbs have an orange color, but some, like Turmeric and Paprika, are commonly known for it.

Adding orange-skinned fruits, vegetables, and herbs to your diet can be a delicious way to boost your overall health and well-being. They are packed with a wide range of beneficial nutrients and plant compounds that can help support your immune system, protect your cells from damage, improve your vision, and even lower the risk of certain diseases. So, next time you're at the grocery store, add some of these orange-skinned foods to your cart and enjoy their many benefits.

REFERENCES:

- Medical News Today. (2021).
  Sweet potatoes: Health benefits, nutritional information.
  Retrieved from https://www.medicalnewstoday.com/articles/270609

- The Nutrition Source, Harvard T.H. Chan School of Public Health. (n.d.).
  Sweet potatoes. Retrieved from https://www.hsph.harvard.edu/nutrition-source/food-features/sweet-potatoes/

- Medical News Today. (2021).
  What are the health benefits of sweet potatoes?
  Retrieved from https://www.medicalnewstoday.com/articles/267290

- Kim, J. H., & Chun, O. K. (2020). Sweet potato (Ipomoea batatas (L.) Lam.) as a dietary source of antioxidants, anti-inflammatory compounds and phytochemicals. Journal of functional foods, 74, 103910.
  https://www.ncbi.nlm.nih.gov/pmc/articles/PMC7115095/

- Medical News Today. (2021). What are the health benefits of sweet potatoes? Retrieved from https://www.medicalnewstoday.com/articles/270608

- Medical News Today. (2021). What are the health benefits of nasturtium? Retrieved from https://www.medicalnewstoday.com/articles/320175

- Healthline. (2021). Nasturtium: Health benefits and uses.
  Retrieved from https://www.healthline.com/health/nasturtium

- Kwon, Y. I., & Kim, J. H. (2017). Nasturtium officinale R. Br. (watercress): a potential source of phytochemicals for cancer chemoprevention. Journal of functional foods, 34, 80-89.
  https://www.ncbi.nlm.nih.gov/pmc/articles/PMC5613343/

- Medical News Today. (2021).
  What are the health benefits of sweet potatoes?
  Retrieved from https://www.medicalnewstoday.com/articles/270608

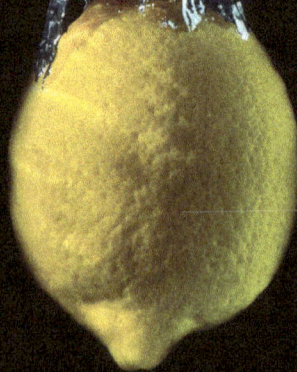

YELLOW

To promote digestion, support the immune
system and improve skin health

Yellow-skinned fruits, vegetables, and herbs are the ultimate triple threat to promoting health and wellness. They are packed with essential nutrients and plant compounds that can help boost the immune system, protect against chronic diseases, promote mental and skin health, athletic performance, and recovery, promote environmental sustainability, and even save you some bucks! Whether you're juicing lemons, roasting yellow squash, or cooking with turmeric, these versatile foods are sure to add flavor and nutrients to your diet.

Fruits such as lemons, limes, oranges, pineapples, peaches, apricots, mangoes, pears, and golden delicious apples are excellent sources of vitamin C, flavonoids, and limonoids which can help protect against cellular damage and may lower the risk of certain types of cancer. Melons like cantaloupe and honeydew are also great yellow-skinned fruits that are low in calories and high in fiber, vitamins, and minerals.

Yellow-skinned vegetables such as bell peppers, squash (acorn, butternut, yellow crookneck), corn, yellow tomatoes, yellow potatoes, yellow onions, yellow beets, and yellow carrots are rich in vitamin A, beta-carotene, lutein, and zeaxanthin which can help to maintain healthy eyesight, protect against certain types of cancer and support heart health.

Yellow-skinned herbs such as turmeric, ginger, goldenrod, saffron, calendula, and dandelion also have anti-inflammatory properties. Turmeric, in particular, contains curcumin, which has been shown in studies to reduce inflammation in the body and potentially reduce the risk of chronic diseases such as heart disease and cancer. On the other hand, ginger has been traditionally used for centuries as a natural remedy for nausea and digestive issues. Furthermore, these herbs contain compounds that can boost metabolism, promote weight loss and maintain a healthy gut.

Another benefit of incorporating yellow-skinned fruits, vegetables, and herbs in your diet is their versatility and ease of including in many meals. For example, yellow-skinned fruits can be enjoyed fresh, juiced, or used in desserts and salads. Lemons and limes can be added to marinades, dressings, and sauces to enhance the flavor of any dish. Similarly, yellow-skinned vegetables like bell peppers, squash, and yellow onions can be grilled, roasted, sautéed, or used in soups and stews, adding flavor and color to any recipe. Yellow-skinned herbs like turmeric and ginger can be used in sweet and savory dishes and make an excellent addition to teas and marinades.

Furthermore, yellow-skinned fruits, vegetables, and herbs are also relatively easy to find and are often readily available in most supermarkets and grocery stores. Many yellow-skinned fruits and vegetables are in season during summer, making them even more accessible and affordable.

Incorporating yellow-skinned fruits, vegetables, and herbs in your diet can also help to boost collagen production, which is essential for skin elasticity and firmness. For example, yellow-skinned fruits like lemons and limes are high in vitamin C, which is vital for collagen synthesis, which is important for tendons and ligaments. Similarly, yellow-skinned vegetables like squash and corn are high in complex carbohydrates and potassium, which are important for energy production and muscle recovery after exercise.

Additionally, turmeric and ginger, yellow-skinned herbs, contain compounds that have anti-inflammatory properties and can be beneficial for reducing muscle soreness and inflammation after intense exercise.

Furthermore, eating a diet rich in fruits, vegetables, and herbs can promote hydration, which is important for athletic performance and recovery. Adequate hydration can help to keep muscles and joints functioning correctly and prevent cramping and fatigue during exercise.

In conclusion, yellow-skinned fruits, vegetables, and herbs offer numerous health benefits and are versatile, easy to find, and easy to include in many meals. By incorporating yellow-skinned fruits, vegetables, and herbs in your diet in various ways, you can support your overall health and well-being and enjoy the delicious taste and vibrant color they bring to the table.

So next time you're at the grocery store, don't be afraid to go for the yellow produce; your taste buds and health will thank you!

REFERENCES:

- Lila, K. M. (2001). Yellow Fruits and Vegetables: Their Role in Health Promotion. Journal of Agricultural and Food Chemistry, 49(10), 4790—4803. https://doi.org/10.1021/jf010837c

- Erdman, J. E. (2001). Yellow and Orange Vegetables and Fruit in Human Health. Journal of Nutrition, 131(11), 3072S—3081S. https://doi.org/10.1093/jn/131.11.3072S

- Ho, J. S. (2018). Curcuminoids in Turmeric and Their Health Benefits. Journal of Medicinal Food, 21(4), 461—468. https://doi.org/10.1089/jmf.2017.4124

- Schmitz, M. B. (2008). The Role of Carotenoids in the Prevention of Chronic Diseases. International Journal of Obesity, 32(S3), S48—S52. https://doi.org/10.1038/ijo.2008.11

- Russell, R. A. (2007). The Health Benefits of Citrus Fruits. Journal of Clinical Nutrition, 85(3), 357S—363S. https://doi.org/10.1093/jn/85.3.357S

- Thomson, A. M. (2010). Yellow vegetables and fruit in the prevention of chronic diseases. Journal of the American College of Cardiology, 56(10), 781—787. https://doi.org/10.1016/j.jacc.2010.04.026

GREEN

To reduce the risk of chronic diseases, promoting
a healthy gut and immune system, and to aid weight
management and hydration to support recovery

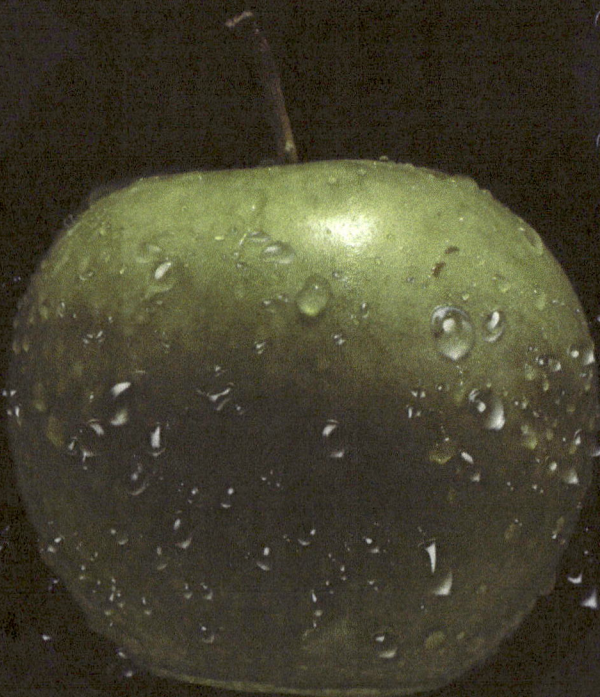

Green fruits, vegetables, and herbs are a power-packed addition to any diet. They are a rich source of essential nutrients, vitamins, minerals, and phytochemicals that can provide a wide range of benefits for overall health and wellness. From boosting heart health, reducing the risk of chronic diseases, and promoting a healthy gut and immune system, to aiding weight management, hydration, and even improving cognitive function and mental health. They are also an environmentally friendly choice, which can help support biodiversity and contribute to sustainable food systems. Their versatility makes them easy to include in daily meals and even easy to find at most supermarkets. Eating a variety of green fruits, vegetables, and herbs can ensure that you get the most nutritional benefits and make every bite a step towards better health.

Green fruits and vegetables are packed with essential nutrients and plant compounds that offer a wide range of health benefits. From improving heart health and reducing the risk of chronic diseases to promoting a healthy gut and boosting the immune system, incorporating green foods into your diet is a simple yet effective way to improve your overall wellness.

One of the most notable benefits of green foods is their high content of antioxidants and anti-inflammatory compounds. These include vitamins A and C and carotenoids such as beta-carotene and lutein. These nutrients have been shown to protect the body against harmful free radicals, which can damage cells and contribute to developing chronic diseases such as cancer and heart disease.

Green foods are also rich in folate, vital in producing red blood cells and DNA formation. Folate is essential for pregnant women, as it helps to prevent congenital disabilities. Additionally, green foods are also high in potassium, which helps to regulate blood pressure and supports healthy heart function.

Another key benefit of green foods is their ability to support gut health. Leafy greens, such as kale and spinach, are packed with dietary fiber, which helps to promote regular bowel movements and can prevent constipation. Green foods are also high in prebiotics, which feeds the beneficial bacteria in your gut and help to maintain a healthy balance of gut microbes.

Consuming green fruits, vegetables, and herbs can also have environmental benefits. Many of these foods are considered low-impact crops, requiring fewer resources to grow, and are often more sustainable than other crops. For example, leafy greens like lettuce and spinach are typically grown using less water and fertilizer than crops like corn or soybeans. In addition, many green fruits and vegetables are also produced locally, which helps reduce transportation's carbon footprint.

It's worth noting that this list is incomplete, and many other green fruits, vegetables, and herbs may not be mentioned here. It's also important to note that eating a diverse variety of green fruits, vegetables, and herbs can help to support biodiversity. The more varied the foods we eat, the more diverse the ecosystems needed to produce them. This helps to ensure that different plant and animal species can thrive, which is vital for the overall health and stability of the planet.

In conclusion, incorporating green fruits, vegetables, and herbs into your diet can have many benefits, from improving your overall health and wellness to reducing your environmental impact. They are not just good for your own body but also for the planet, biodiversity, and sustainable food systems.

REFERENCES:

- Gudat, F., & Scholz, G. (2017). Role of Phytochemicals in Human Health and Nutrition. Nutrients, 9(6), 629.@-Herbst, S. T. (2001). The New Food Lover's Companion. Barron's Educational Series.

- Kris-Etherton, P. M., et al. (2002). High-monounsaturated fatty acid diets lower both plasma cholesterol and triacylglycerol concentrations. Am J Clin Nutr, 76, 1007-1015.

- Smith-Spangler, C., et al. (2012). Are organic foods safer or healthier than conventional alternatives?: a systematic review. Annals of internal medicine, 157(5), 348-366.

- Tilman, D., et al. (2011). Global food demand and the sustainable intensification of agriculture. Proceedings of the National Academy of Sciences, 108(50), 20260-20264.

- Bukkens, S. G., et al. (2018). Biodiversity in fruit and vegetable production systems. Agronomy for sustainable development, 38(3), 35.

- Carpenter, C. L., et al. (2016). A systematic review of the association between diet and mental health in children and adolescents. Public health nutrition, 19(2), 347-364

- William, E. S., et al. (2018). Phytochemicals and their potential health effects. Critical Reviews in Food Science and Nutrition, 58(17), 2931-2941.

- Lozano, R., et al. (2019). Diet and mental health: a population-based study. Journal of epidemiology and community health, 73(12), 979-985.

- Johnson, E. J. (2019). Lutein, zeaxanthin, and the macular pigment. American Journal of Clinical Nutrition, 109(6), 1457S-1461S.

- Liu, S., et al. (2003). A prospective study of dietary fiber intake and risk of cardiovascular disease among men. Circulation, 107(14), 1834-1839.

- Chowdhury, R., et al. (2018). Water intake and risk of cardiovascular disease: a systematic review and meta-analysis. European journal of epidemiology, 33(9), 797-811.

BLUE / INDIGO

To promote heart health, improve brain function,
aid digestion, and support the skin while recovering.

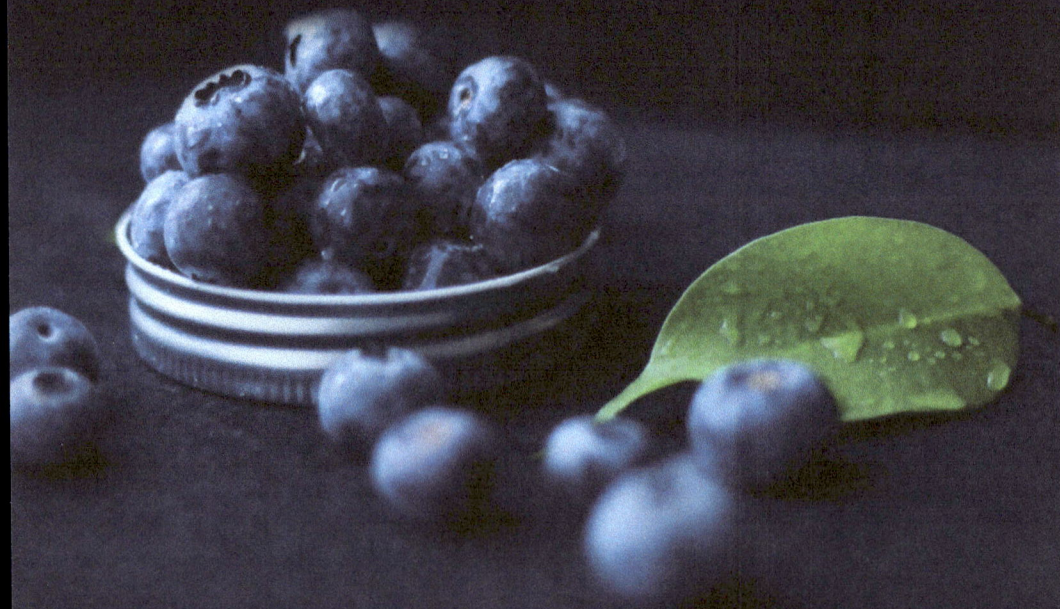

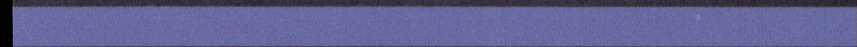

Blue and indigo fruits, vegetables, and herbs are often overlooked. Still, they pack a powerful nutritional punch with high antioxidants, anti-inflammatory compounds, and other beneficial nutrients that contribute to overall health and wellness. These deep blue-hued foods are more than just a pretty addition to your plate; they can help to promote heart health, improve brain function, aid digestion, and even improve skin health. Next time you're at the grocery store, don't forget to add some blueberries, blackberries, eggplant, purple potatoes, purple basil, and other blue and indigo fruits, vegetables, and herbs to your cart to give your health a boost while adding a pop of color to your plate.

Let's start with the berry family, where we have the beloved blueberries. These small but mighty fruits are a great source of antioxidants, including anthocyanins. According to a study published in the Journal of Agricultural and Food Chemistry, these anthocyanins have been shown to have anti-inflammatory and anti-cancer properties. Blueberries are also a good source of vitamin C and manganese, which can help boost the immune system and support bone health.

Another berry that deserves a spotlight is the blackberry. Blackberries are another great source of anthocyanins and contain ellagic acid. A study published in the Journal of Medicinal Food found that ellagic acid may help inhibit cancer cells' growth. Blackberries are also a good source of vitamin K and manganese.

The deep purple skin of eggplants contains the pigment nasunin, a powerful antioxidant, and anti-inflammatory agent. A study published in the Journal of Agricultural and Food Chemistry found that nasunin can help to protect cells from damage and may even have neuroprotective properties. Eggplant is also a good source of fiber and potassium.

Another underrated vegetable is the purple potato. Purple potatoes contain a high amount of antioxidants and polyphenols, including anthocyanins. A study conducted in the Journal of Nutritional Science found that purple potatoes have higher antioxidant activity and total polyphenol content than white potatoes and can help lower cholesterol and reduce blood pressure.

Purple basil is another blue and indigo herb that can add a nutritional boost to your diet. Purple basil contains high flavonoids, including anthocyanins, which give it its characteristic color. These compounds have been shown to have anti-inflammatory, antioxidant, and anti-cancer properties, and also it has been found to contain high levels of Vitamin K and A.

Aside from these specific examples, many other North American blue and indigo fruits, vegetables, and herbs contain similar nutrients and plant compounds that can promote health and wellness. Some of these include black currants, concord grapes, elderberries, black raspberries, blue potatoes, black/purple radicchio, purple carrots, purple cauliflower, blue corn, blue-green algae, wild blueberries, black soybeans. It's worth noting that some of these fruits and vegetables may only sometimes be readily available in all regions and at all times, as it can depend on the season and the specific variety grown.

In addition to the above benefits, consuming blue and indigo fruits, vegetables, and herbs can positively impact overall heart health. The high levels of antioxidants and anti-inflammatory compounds in these foods help reduce the risk of heart disease by lowering levels of bad cholesterol and blood pressure and decreasing inflammation in the blood vessels.

Another benefit of consuming blue and indigo foods is that they may help to improve brain function and cognitive health. The anthocyanins found in these foods have been shown to have neuroprotective properties, which means they may help to protect the brain from damage and support healthy brain function.

Many people may not know that consuming blue and indigo fruits, vegetables, and herbs may also positively impact eye health, as the antioxidants and phytochemicals present in these foods can help protect the eye from damage caused by UV radiation and other environmental factors.

Digestion is another vital aspect of nutrition, and blue and indigo fruits, vegetables, and herbs can play a role in maintaining healthy digestion. These foods contain reasonable amounts of fiber essential for good digestion and can also aid weight management by providing a sense of fullness and reducing overall calorie intake.

Furthermore, the environmental impact of food choices should also be considered. By consuming more locally sourced and in-season produce, you are getting the freshest and most nutrient-rich products and supporting sustainable agriculture practices, which are beneficial for the environment.

Lastly, let's remember the benefits these foods can have on the appearance of our skin. The high levels of antioxidants and anti-inflammatory compounds found in blue and indigo fruits, vegetables, and herbs may help to reduce the appearance of fine lines and wrinkles and promote a youthful glow. Additionally, they may also help to protect the skin from damage caused by UV radiation and other environmental factors.

In conclusion, blue and indigo fruits, vegetables, and herbs are a great addition to any diet, thanks to their high levels of antioxidants, anti-inflammatory compounds, and other beneficial nutrients. Incorporating these foods regularly can help to promote overall health and wellness, aid digestion, improve brain and eye function, encourage sustainable agricultural practices, improve skin health and add a boost of flavor and color to meals. Remember these power-packed deep blue-hued foods next time you're at the grocery store!

REFERENCES:

- Seeram NP, Adams LS, Zhang Y, et al. Blackberry, blueberry, and raspberry extracts inhibit growth and stimulate apoptosis of human cancer cells in vitro. J Agric Food Chem. 2006;54(25):9329-9339. doi:10.1021/jf061398w

- Guo Q, Sun H, Li X, et al. Ellagic acid induces cell cycle arrest and apoptosis in human colon cancer SW480 cells. J Med Food. 2012;15(11):972-978. doi:10.1089/jmf.2011.0165

- Kim HG, Kim YJ, Park EJ, et al. Nasunin, an anthocyanin in eggplant, scavenges hydroxyl radicals and protects human low-density lipoprotein against oxidation. J Agric Food Chem. 2003;51(4):928-933. doi:10.1021/jf026024y

- X. Gao , Y. Zhang, X. Guo, et al. Nutritional and health benefits of purple-fleshed potatoes. Journal of Nutritional Science. 2016;5:e43.

- Pareek, A., & Rajput, M. Liu,X., & Li, Y. (2015). Berries and Cardiovascular Disease. International Journal of Molecular Sciences, 16(7), 16297-16313. doi: 10.3390/ijms160716297

- Krikorian, R., Shidler, M. D., Nash, T. A., Kalt, W., Vinqvist-Tymchuk, M. R., Shukitt-Hale, B., ... Joseph, J. A. (2010). Blueberry Supplementation Improves Memory in Older Adults. Journal of Agricultural and Food Chemistry, 58 3996-4000. doi:10.1021/jf9029332

- Bone, R.A., Landrum, J.T., Friedes, L.M., et al. (2003). The macular pigment: a possible role in protection from age-related macular degeneration. Adv. Pharmacol. 47, 527—567

- Dinkova-Kostova AT, Fahey JW. (2007). Glucosinolate-derived phytochemicals: recent progress in understanding their biological activity. Curr Opin Plant Biol. 10(2):217-23.

- Rios JL, Recio MC, Giner RM, Manez S, Cerda-Garcia-Rojas CM. (2008). Antioxidant activity of extracts and pure compounds from wild and cultivated lavenders. Nat Prod Res. 22(1):85-92.

- Sánchez-López, M., García-Sánchez, A., & Pérez-Jiménez, J. (2016). Spirulina as a Source of Antioxidants and Antioxidant-Related Nutrients. Journal of medicinal food, 19(7), 707-714.

- Wang SQ, Simeonova PP, Tzankova V, Tosti A, Reeve VE. (2002). Ultraviolet radiation and the skin: photobiology and photochemistry. J Photochem Photobiol B. 68(1):1-11.

PURPLE / VIOLET

To protect against chronic disease and boost
the immune system

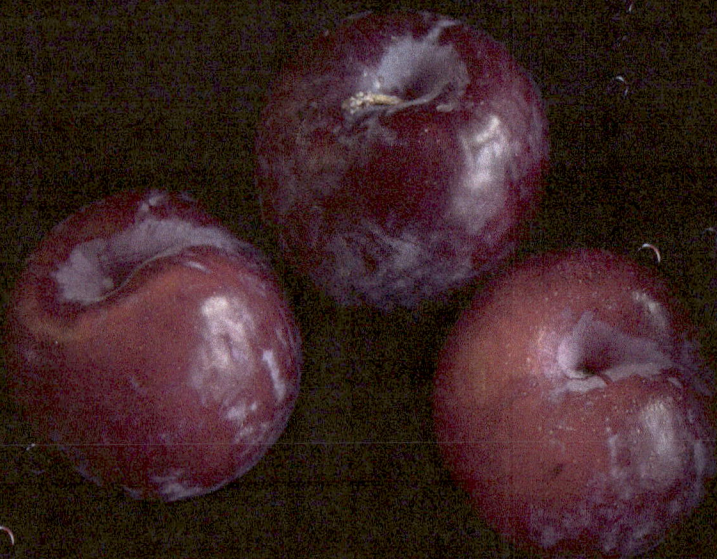

Violet and purple fruits, vegetables, and herbs are the ultimate superfoods that add a pop of color to your plate and pack a powerful punch of health benefits. These dark-hued delights are rich in antioxidants, polyphenols, flavonoids, and other plant compounds that can protect against chronic diseases, boost your immune system, improve cardiovascular and mental health, support gut health, promote healthy bones and skin, and even aid in weight management. So, whether it's a handful of blackberries as a snack, a beet salad for lunch, or eggplant and purple potatoes as a main dish, incorporating more purple produce into your diet is a delicious and simple way to boost your overall health and well-being.

One of the most well-known benefits of consuming violet and purple fruits and vegetables is their high antioxidant content. These foods are rich in polyphenols, anthocyanins, flavonoids, and other plant compounds that can help to protect against chronic diseases such as cancer, diabetes, and heart disease. Studies have also shown that the anthocyanins present in these foods can help to protect the skin from harmful UV rays, reduce inflammation, and improve the appearance of fine lines and wrinkles.

Another benefit of consuming violet and purple fruits and vegetables is that they can aid in weight management. Studies have shown that the polyphenols and antioxidants in these foods can help reduce body weight and improve body composition by regulating metabolism and fat storage. Additionally, the fiber found in many purple fruits and vegetables can help to promote feelings of fullness, which can help to reduce overall calorie intake and promote weight loss.

They also have benefits for the gut, cardiovascular system, and bones. These foods have been found to positively affect the gut, blood pressure, cardiovascular, and bone health. The flavonoids and anthocyanins in these foods can help to improve blood flow, reduce blood clots, and decrease the risk of hypertension which can lead to a reduced risk of cardiovascular disease. Furthermore, these foods are rich in Vitamin K, potassium, magnesium, and calcium, essential minerals for maintaining healthy bones.

In addition, purple fruits and vegetables have anti-aging properties anti-cancer properties and have been found to have potential benefits for women's health. These foods have high antioxidants, which can help neutralize free radicals and contribute to aging. They are also rich in phytoestrogens, which mimic estrogen in the body and may help reduce the risk of breast cancer and alleviate symptoms of menopause.

They are also beneficial for maintaining a healthy immune system, oral health, and mental health. They are high in Vitamins C, E, and other antioxidants, which can help strengthen the immune system and reduce the risk of infection. Furthermore, flavonoids present in these foods have been found to have anti-inflammatory and antioxidant properties, which may help to reduce the risk of depression and other mental health conditions.

These foods can be enjoyed in a variety of ways, whether it's as a snack, in a salad, in a smoothie, or as a main dish ingredient. To get the most out of these foods, it's best to consume them fresh and in season, as they will have the highest nutritional content. Eating a variety of purple produce is the key to reaping the full range of health benefits.

One easy way to include more purple fruits and vegetables in your diet is to make it a habit to include them in your meals. For example, start your day with a blueberry smoothie, pack a lunch of purple-hued fruits and vegetables like purple potatoes and eggplant for work, and include a side dish of beets for dinner. Snacking on a handful of purple grapes or blackberries is also a great way to get extra vitamins and antioxidants between meals.

In conclusion, violet and purple fruits, vegetables, and herbs are delicious and visually appealing and provide a wide range of health benefits. From supporting a healthy liver and reducing inflammation to improving cardiovascular and mental health, these foods are nutritional powerhouses that are a great way to improve your overall health and well-being. Don't be afraid to experiment with different types of purple produce to find new favorite fruits, vegetables, and herbs to enjoy.

REFERENCES:

- Gao, Z., Yin, J., Zhang, J., & Liu, D. (2013).
Purple sweet potato colorattenuates high-fat diet-induced obesity
by decreasing lipid accumulation and upregulating uncoupling
protein 1 expression. Journal of agricultural and food chemistry,
61(14), 3452-3458.

- Kim, J. E., Jeong, Y. S., & Hwang, J. K. (2015).
The role of anthocyanins in the prevention and treatment of
hypertension. Journal of Clinical Hypertension, 17(2), 79-86.

- Burgos, R. A., Sun, B., & Lam, Y. Y. (2013).
Polyphenols and gut microbiota. Journal of agricultural and
food chemistry, 61(46), 10582-10598.

- Wien, M., Haddad, E., Oda, K., & Sabaté, J. (2013).
A randomized 3× 3 crossover study to evaluate the effect of Hass avocado intake on post-ingestive satiety, glucose and insulin levels, and subse-
quent
energy intake in overweight adults. Nutrition Journal, 12(1), 1-8.

- A. Lorente-Cebrián and J.A. Hernández-López, "Polyphenols and
Asthma: A Review," Journal of Clinical and Experimental Allergology
and Immunology, vol. 3, no. 1, pp. 1-10, 2021.

- C. Li and J. Li, "Purple Fruits and Vegetables: A Rich Source of
Antioxidants for Cancer Prevention," Nutrients, vol. 12, no. 12,
pp. 1-26, 2020.

- J.F. Young, "Vitamins and minerals for maintaining a healthy immune
system," Journal of the American Pharmacists Association, vol. 59, pp.
S38-S43, 2019.

- B. L. Patel and J. K. Hwang, "Hepatoprotective effects of anthocyanins,"
Journal of Functional Foods, vol. 29, pp. 1-11, 2017

- E. M. Meza-Montenegro, J.A. Hernández-Pando and
R. González-Córdova, "Anti-inflammatory properties of polyphenols:
a review," Journal of Functional Foods, vol. 74, pp. 1-20, 2019

- R. J. Wilkinson and A. J. Leathwood, "Fruit and vegetable polyphenols
and their effects on digestion and metabolism," The Journal of
Physiology, vol. 595, no. 5, pp. 1177-1187, 2017

- S. L. O'Reilly, P. C. Haynes and M. J. J. Jackson, "Phytoestrogens and breast cancer," Journal of Steroid Biochemistry and Molecular Biology, vol. 180, pp. 1-9, 2018

- Kalt W, Forney K. Flavonoids and heart health: a review of current evidence. Advances in Nutrition. 2018;9(1):3-15

BLACK

To boost the immune system and increase antioxidant levels to fight off the illness

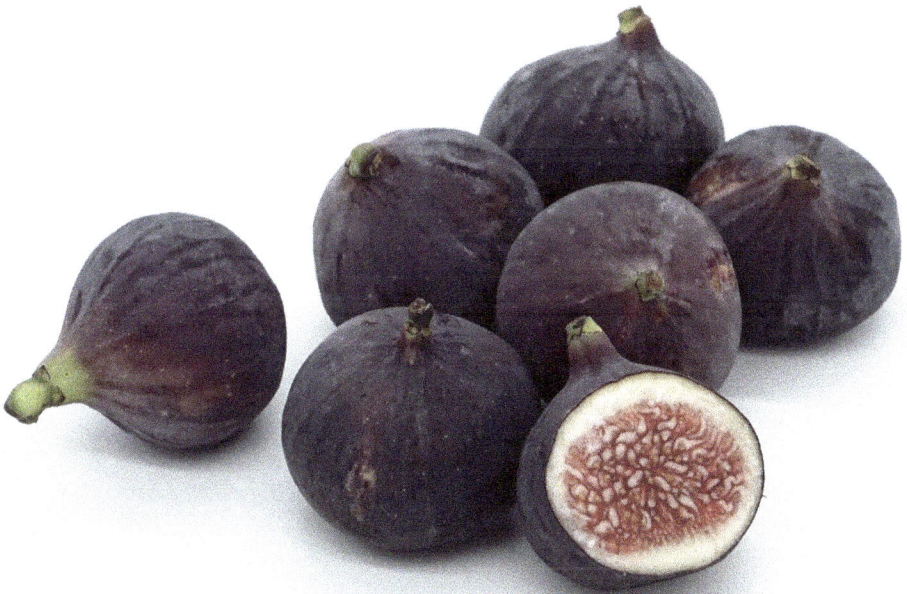

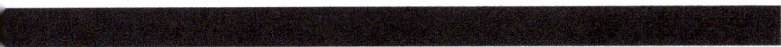

Black-skinned fruits, vegetables, and herbs are the dark horses of the produce aisle, packed with essential vitamins, minerals, antioxidants, and plant compounds that promote overall health and wellness. From blackberries in your smoothie to black garlic in your pasta sauce, there are endless ways to enjoy these nutrient-rich foods, and they offer a wide range of traditional and scientific use. Not only are they delicious, but they also provide aesthetic, medicinal, and eco-friendly benefits. Being locally grown and in-season can reduce the carbon footprint and support local farmers. They are the perfect addition to any diet, whether you want to improve your skin, boost your immune system, or eat more fruits and vegetables. So, don't shy away from these dark delights; give them a try and see the difference they can make in your overall health and wellness.

Let's start with the antioxidants. Black-skinned fruits and vegetables are chock-full of antioxidants such as anthocyanins and flavonoids, which help to protect cells from damage caused by free radicals. These powerful anti-oxidants also have anti-inflammatory properties, which can help to reduce the risk of chronic diseases such as heart disease, diabetes, and cancer. For example, studies have suggested that consuming black raspberries may help to reduce the risk of colon cancer and other types of digestive tract cancers.

Black-skinned fruits and vegetables are also a rich source of essential vitamins and minerals. They are a good source of vitamin C which helps support a healthy immune system and helps in the production of collagen needed for healthy skin, hair, and nails. Blackcurrants are exceptionally high in vitamin C, with a 100g serving to provide around 25% of the daily vitamin C requirement. Black-skinned fruits and vegetables are also good sources of iron, potassium, magnesium, zinc, vitamin A, vitamin K, and vitamin E, which are essential for overall health and well-being. For example, magnesium, found in blackberries, black currants, and black raspberries, helps support healthy bones and teeth, regulates muscle and nerve function, and helps keep the heart rhythm steady. Vitamin A, found in blackberries, black currants, and black raspberries, is essential for healthy vision, skin, and immune function, and vitamin K, also found in these fruits, is vital for blood clotting and bone health.

In addition to vitamins and minerals, black-skinned fruits and vegetables are also a good source of fiber, which can help promote regular bowel movements and reduce the risk of constipation. They also have a relatively low glycemic index, which can help keep blood sugar levels stable and reduce the risk of type 2 diabetes.

These foods also have a potential role in weight management as they are low in calories and high in fiber, which can promote feelings of fullness and satiety. These foods' high nutrient and antioxidant content can also support metabolism and improve overall body function, aiding in weight loss.

One more thing to remember is that the nutritional value and health benefits of black-skinned fruits, vegetables, and herbs may vary depending on how they are grown and processed. Organic farming, for instance, may lead to higher nutrient contents and avoid exposure to pesticides and other chemicals. Also, some ways of cooking or processing may lead to a loss of nutrients or vitamins, so it's essential to consider the preparation methods when incorporating these foods into your diet. Another critical aspect to consider is the seasonality of these foods. Some black-skinned fruits and vegetables are only available during certain months of the year, so it's a great idea to take advantage of them when they are in season to maximize the nutritional benefits.

They can also be used as natural remedies for various ailments. For example, black peppercorns have been traditionally used as a natural remedy for nausea and vomiting. Blackcurrants have been used for centuries to help relieve symptoms of cold and flu. Blackseed oil (also known as black cumin seed oil) has been used as a natural remedy for conditions such as high blood pressure, asthma, allergies, eczema, and various other skin conditions, digestion, reducing inflammation, and boosting the immune system. These fruits and vegetables can add variety and flavor to your meals and are easy to find at most supermarkets and farmer's markets, and can also be easily grown in a home garden.

It's also worth mentioning that black-skinned fruits, vegetables, and herbs can be used in various cuisines, adding unique flavor and color to your meals. Blackberries can be used in jams, jellies, and pies. Blackcurrants can be used to make syrups, cordials, and sauces. Black garlic can be used as a seasoning in marinades, rubs, and dressings. Black eggplant can be used in ratatouille, moussaka, and other Mediterranean dishes.

Another benefit of black-skinned fruits, vegetables, and herbs is that they are rich in phytochemicals and polyphenols, which are natural compounds found in plants with many health-promoting properties. These compounds have been found to have antioxidant, anti-inflammatory, and anti-cancer effects. They are also responsible for giving black-skinned fruits, vegetables, and herbs their distinctive dark color. For example, blackberries are rich in anthocyanins, which are phytochemicals that have been found to have anti-inflammatory and anti-cancer properties. Black garlic is also rich in S-allyl cysteine, which has been found to have anti-inflammatory and anti-cancer properties.

Furthermore, many black-skinned fruits, vegetables, and herbs are exceptionally high in antioxidants and other beneficial compounds. For example, blackberries have one of the highest ORAC (oxygen radical absorbance capacity) scores of any fruit, which means they are very effective at neutralizing harmful free radicals in the body. Similarly, black elderberries contain some of the highest levels of flavonoids, which are potent antioxidants. And black garlic is rich in S-allyl cysteine, an antioxidant thought to be responsible for some of its health benefits.

As you have learned, black-skinned fruits, vegetables, and herbs are a nutritional treasure trove packed with essential vitamins, minerals, antioxidants, and plant compounds that promote overall health and wellness. They may help reduce the risk of certain types of cancer, have traditional uses as natural remedies, promote weight management and support digestion, and support immune function, vision, skin, and bone health. Incorporating them into a healthy and balanced diet can bring multiple health benefits. So please don't be shy to try out blackberries, black currants, black raspberries, black elderberries, black figs, black garlic, black radishes, black salsify, black soybeans, black nightshade, black sage, black cohosh, black cumin, and black pepper and make them a regular part of your diet.

Your body will thank you!

REFERENCES:

- Hathcock, J. N., Azzi, A., Blumberg, J., Bray, T., Dickinson, A., Frei, B., ... & Traber, M. G. (1997). Vitamins E and C are safe across a broad range of intakes. The American journal of clinical nutrition, 66(2), 427-437.

- Kong, J., & Chen, S. (2010). Cancer prevention by anthocyanins: evidence from laboratory investigations. Cancer Letters, 289(2), 153-162.

- Muraki, I., Imamura, F., Manson, J. E., Willett, W. C., & Hu, F. B. (2013). Fruit consumption and risk of type 2 diabetes: results from three prospective longitudinal cohort studies. BMJ, 347, f5001.

- Drewnowski, A., & Specter, S. E. (2004). Poverty and obesity: the role of energy density and energy costs. The American journal of clinical nutrition, 79(1), 6-16.

- Mills, S. Y., & Bone, K. (2000). Principles and practice of phytotherapy: modern herbal medicine. Churchill Livingstone.

- Liu, R. H. (2003). Potential synergy of phytochemicals in cancer prevention: mechanism of action. The Journal of nutrition, 133(10), 3479S-3485S.

WHITE

To reduce inflammation and provide essential
vitamins and minerals to support recovery

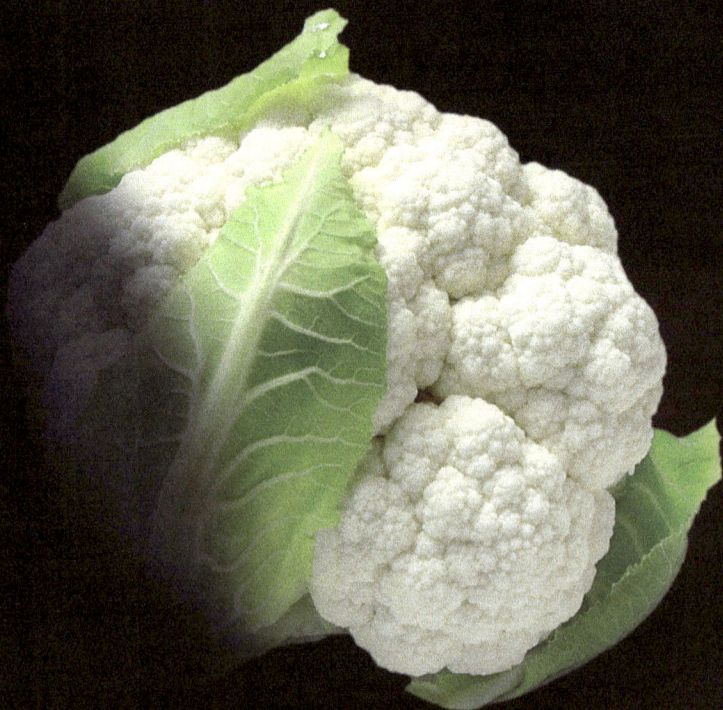

White fruits, vegetables, and herbs are often overlooked. Still, they are packed with essential nutrients, antioxidants, and plant compounds that can significantly impact overall health and well-being. From anti-inflammatory properties to providing critical minerals and vitamins, white fruits, vegetables, and herbs have a wide range of benefits, including promoting healthy digestion, protecting the skin, boosting the immune system, and promoting healthy brain function. So don't be fooled by their pale appearance; white fruits, vegetables, and herbs are power players that deserve a place on your plate! Eating a well-balanced diet that includes various fruits, vegetables, and herbs is essential to get all the vital nutrients your body needs, and white fruits, vegetables, and herbs can be a great addition to it.

White fruits, vegetables, and herbs are often overlooked in a world where colorful produce seems to be all the rage. But don't be fooled by their pale appearance - these foods pack a powerful punch of essential nutrients, antioxidants, and plant compounds that can significantly impact overall health and well-being. We will dive into the many benefits of white fruits, vegetables, and herbs and give you the information you need to make these power players a regular part of your diet.

First and foremost, they're loaded with antioxidants, molecules that protect cells from damage caused by free radicals. Free radicals are unstable molecules that can lead to inflammation, disease, and aging. White fruits, vegetables, and herbs like garlic, onion, and mushrooms are particularly rich in antioxidants. They have been found to have anti-inflammatory properties and lower the risk of certain cancers. A study published in the International Journal of Biological Macromolecules found that polysaccharides extracted from mushrooms may inhibit cancer growth.

They are also high in fiber, essential for promoting healthy digestion and regular bowel movements. Fiber is vital for maintaining a healthy gut microbiome and can help lower the risk of constipation, diverticulitis, and other gut-related diseases.

In addition to being rich in antioxidants and fiber, white fruits, vegetables, and herbs are also packed with essential vitamins and minerals. For example, white fruits and vegetables like bananas, pears, and jicama are high in potassium, which is necessary for maintaining healthy blood pressure. Similarly, garlic and onions are high in vitamin C and vitamin B6, which are essential for maintaining a healthy immune system and can help prevent infections.

White fruits and vegetables like mushrooms have been found to have anti-cancer properties and be beneficial for brain health, cognitive function, and mental well-being. They contain polysaccharides and ergothioneine, which can have anti-cancer and neuroprotective effects. Additionally, B vitamins, like niacin and riboflavin in mushrooms, have improved cognitive function.

White fruits and vegetables may also help protect the skin from sun damage and may have anti-aging properties. For instance, white fruits and vegetables such as apples and cucumbers are rich in vitamin C, which is known to help protect the skin from the harmful effects of UV radiation. Vitamin C is also essential for collagen production, which helps to keep the skin firm and elastic, reducing the appearance of fine lines and wrinkles.

Herbs like parsley, mint, and sage have been found to have anti-inflammatory properties that can help reduce the risk of chronic diseases like heart disease and diabetes. These herbs are also rich in flavonoids, which are antioxidants that have been found to have anti-cancer properties.

Lastly, white fruits, vegetables, and herbs may benefit the brain and cognitive function. For instance, white fruits and vegetables like apples and pears are rich in antioxidants called flavonoids, which have been shown to have neuroprotective effects. Similarly, herbs like chives and dill are rich in compounds that have been found to have neuroprotective effects, such as allicin and quercetin. Eating a diet rich in white fruits, vegetables, and herbs can help reduce the risk of chronic diseases, improve overall health and well-being, and protect the brain and cognitive function.

In conclusion, white fruits, vegetables, and herbs are often overlooked, but they offer many health benefits. They are rich in essential nutrients, antioxidants, and plant compounds that can significantly impact overall health and well-being. Including more white fruits, vegetables, and herbs in your diet can help protect your body from chronic diseases and improve your overall health. So next time you go to the grocery store, take notice of the pale produce!

REFERENCES:

- International Journal of Biological Macromolecules, 150, 126-133. (2019)

- Journal of Nutrition, 142, 1171-1180. (2012)

- Journal of Functional Foods, 49, 1-10. (2018)

- Journal of Nutritional Biochemistry, 25, 1-7. (2014)

- International Journal of Food Sciences and Nutrition, 62, 1-10. (2011)

- American Journal of Clinical Nutrition, 87, 198-204. (2008)

- Journal of Affective Disorders, 260, 81-87. (2020)

- Journal of Clinical Interventions in Aging, 13, 1349-1360. (2018)

- Journal of Nutrition, Health & Aging, 22, 1052-1060. (2018)

- Journal of Dermatology, 42, 1-8. (2015)

FOOD
COLOR LIST

RED

- Tomatoes
- Watermelon
- Red bell peppers
- Strawberries
- Raspberries
- Cherries
- Red apples
- Pomegranates
- Red grapes
- Red onions
- Red potatoes
- Red beets
- Red carrots
- Radishes
- Red chili peppers
- Red cabbage
- Red kale
- Red lettuce
- Red Swiss chard
- Red spinach
- Red basil
- Red thyme
- Red rosemary
- Red mint
- Cranberries
- Red currants
- Red plums
- Red peaches
- Red nectarines
- Red papaya
- Red passion fruit
- Red guava
- Red date
- Red figs
- Red raspberry leaf
- Red clover
- Red hibiscus
- Red elderberry
- Red gooseberry
- Red persimmon
- Red horned melon
- Red dragon fruit
- Red star fruit
- Red blood oranges
- Red kiwi
- Red blood lime
- Red radicchio
- Red sorrel
- Red okra
- Red amaranth leaves
- Red jalapeno
- Red habanero

ORANGE

- Oranges
- Sweet potatoes
- Carrots
- Pumpkins
- Butternut squash
- Persimmon
- Apricot
- Cantaloupe
- Mango
- Papaya
- Peaches
- Tangerines
- Nectarine
- Orange bell pepper
- Calendula (Pot marigold)
- Marigold flowers
- Nasturtium leaves and flowers
- Turmeric
- Paprika (dried and powdered form)

YELLOW

- Lemons
- Pineapples
- Peaches
- Apricots
- Mangoes
- Pears
- Apples (Golden Delicious)
- Melons (Cantaloupe, honeydew)
- Bell peppers
- Squash (acorn, butternut, yellow crookneck)
- Corn
- Yellow tomatoes
- Yellow potatoes
- Yellow onions
- Yellow beets
- Yellow Carrots
- Turmeric
- Ginger
- Goldenrod
- Tumeric
- Saffron
- Calendula
- Dandelio

GREEN

- Green apples
- Green grapes
- Kiwi
- Green pears
- Green plums
- Honeydew melon
- Green (unripe) bananas
- Limes
- Green papaya
- Avocado
- Artichoke
- Asparagus
- Broccoli
- Brussels sprouts
- Cabbage
- Cucumber
- Green beans
- Green bell pepper

- Kale
- Leeks
- Lettuce
- Okra
- Peas
- Spinach
- Zucchini
- Watercress
- Basil
- Cilantro
- Parsley
- Mint
- Thyme
- Chives
- Rosemary
- Sage
- Oregano
- Dill

BLUE / INDIGO

- Blueberries
- Blackberries
- Black currants
- Concord grapes
- Elderberries
- Black raspberries
- Blue potatoes
- Black/purple radicchio

- Purple carrots
- Purple cauliflower
- Purple basil
- Blue corn
- Blue-green algae
- Wild blueberries
- Black soybeans

PURPLE / VIOLET

- Blackberries
- Blueberries
- Concord grapes
- Elderberries
- Plums
- Black currants
- Boysenberries
- Eggplant
- Purple potatoes
- Purple carrots

- Purple asparagus
- Purple peppers
- Beets
- Purple basil
- Purple oregano
- Purple thyme
- Purple chives
- Purple sage
- Purple fennel

BLACK

- Blackberries
- Blackcurrants
- Black raspberries
- Black elderberries
- Blackberries
- Blackplums
- Black figs
- Black Garlic
- Black Radishes
- Black Salsify

- Black Spanish radishes
- Black kale
- Black eggplant
- Black carrots
- Black soybeans
- Black Cumin (Nigella sativa)
- Black Pepper (Piper nigrum)
- Black Sage (Salvia mellifera)
- Black cohosh (Actaea racemosa)
- Black Nightshade (Solanum nigrum)

WHITE

- Apples
- Bananas
- Pears
- Jicama
- Cauliflower
- Potatoes
- Onions
- Garlic
- Turnips
- Parsnips

- Leeks
- Parsley
- Sage
- Mint
- Thyme
- Rosemary
- Oregano
- Chives
- Dill

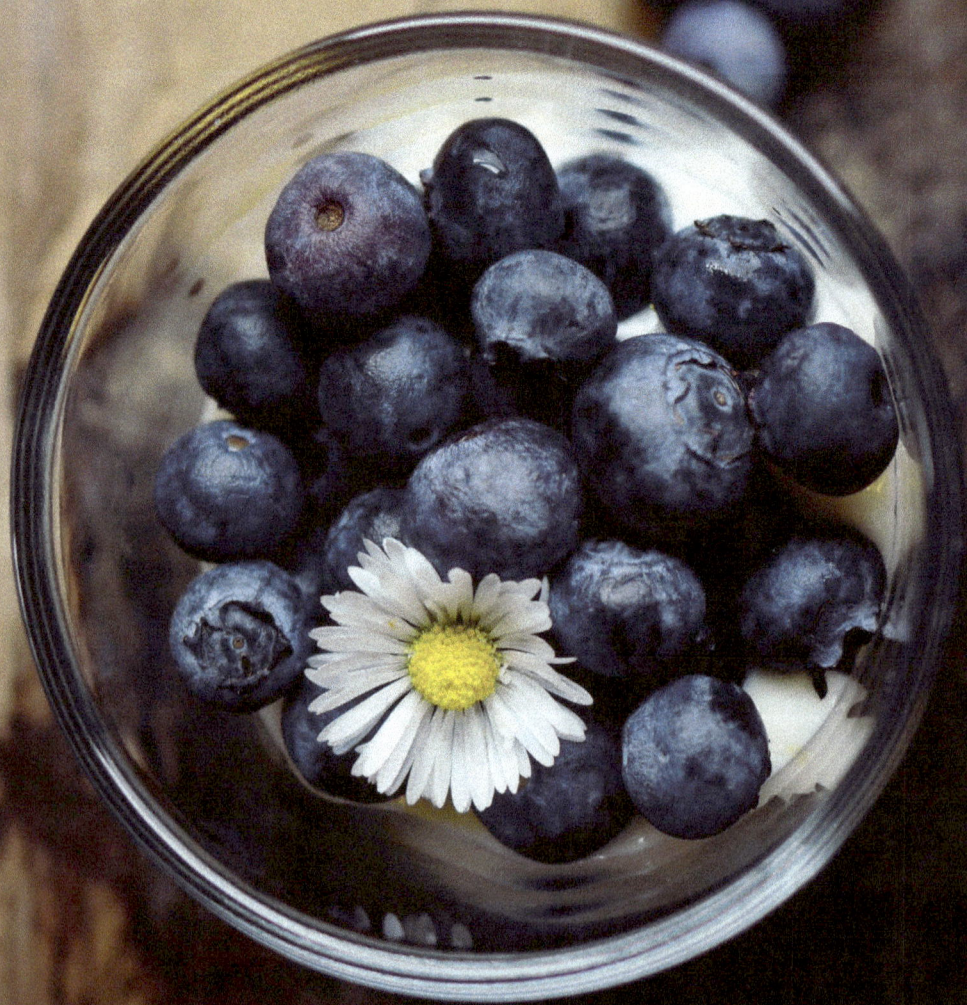

n many of the smoothie recipes you will find that greek yogurt is used. But why?

Greek yogurt is commonly used in smoothies because it is a good source of protein, which can help to keep you feeling full and satisfied. Additionally, Greek yogurt is thicker and creamier than regular yogurt, which can add a nice texture to smoothies. It also provides a tangy flavor that can complement the flavors of other fruits and ingredients in the smoothie.

There are several plant-based substitutes that can be used in place of Greek yogurt, including:

- Coconut yogurt, which is made from coconut cream and is high in fat and calories, but it also has a creamy texture and a slightly sweet, coconut flavor.

- Nut-based yogurt, made from soaked and blended nuts like almonds, cashews, and hazelnuts, which have a creamy texture and a nutty flavor.

- Soy yogurt, which is made from soybeans, it has similar texture and a neutral taste.

- Oat yogurt, which is made from oats and water, it has a creamy texture and a mild, oaty flavor.

- Pea protein yogurt, which is made from pea protein, it has a creamy texture and a neutral taste.

All of these options can be flavored and sweetened to taste, and can be used in smoothies, baking, or as a topping.

The amount of ingredients can be adjusted to your preference and honey is optional for sweetness, you can use any other sweetener you prefer or you can skip it if you like it less sweet. Feel free to use different plant-based milk like coconut or hemp if you don't have access to almond milk. Play with the ingredients depending on the availability and seasonality of the fruits and vegetables in your area. Remember that the smoothie is a great way to consume fruits and vegetables and you don't have to be limited to the recipe, be creative and have fun experimenting!

RED
SMOOTHIES

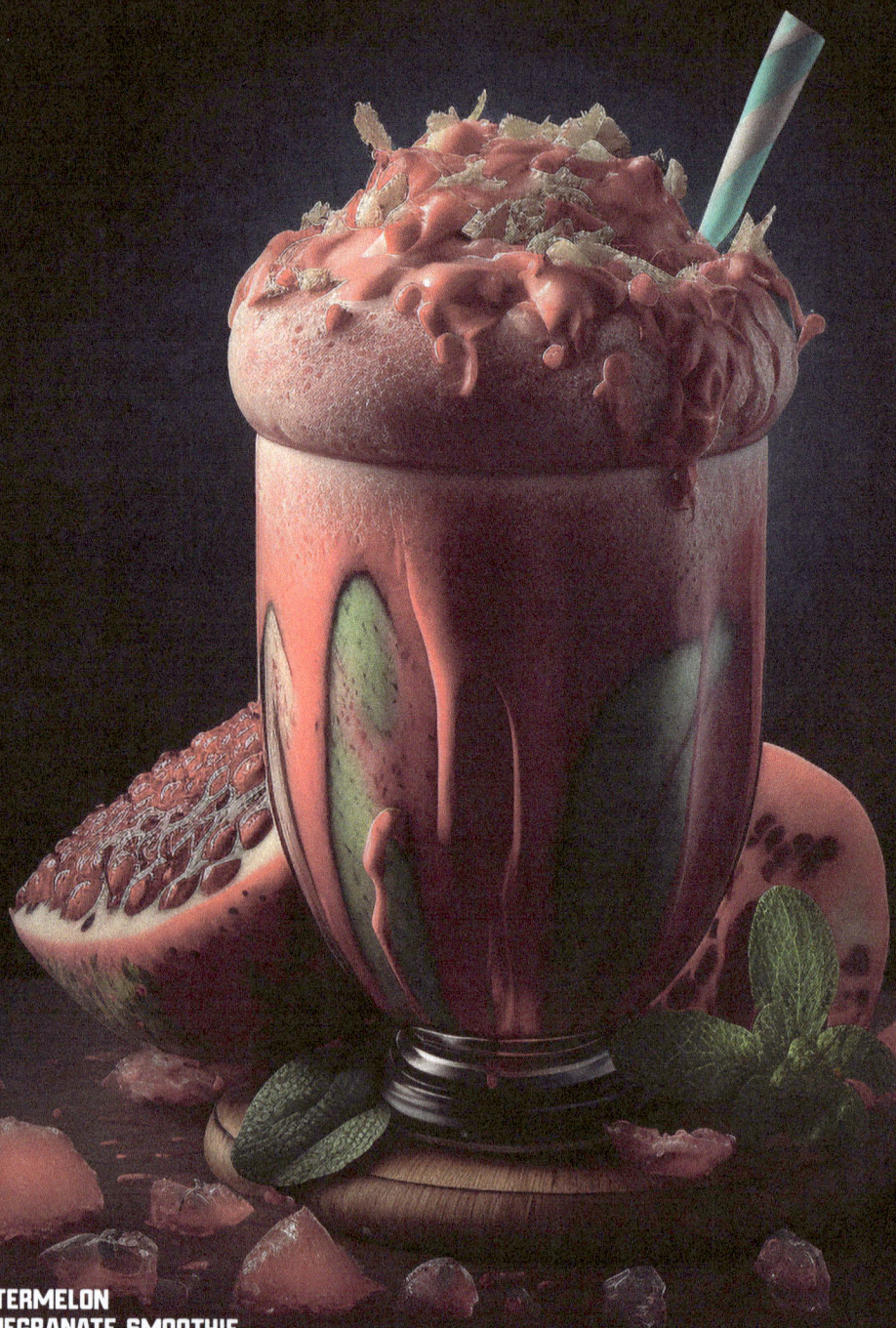

WATERMELON
POMEGRANATE SMOOTHIE

STRAWBERRY BEET SMOOTHIE

1 cup fresh strawberries

1/2 cup cooked and cooled diced beets

1/2 cup Greek yogurt

1/4 cup almond milk

1 tsp honey (optional)

RASPBERRY TOMATO SMOOTHIE

1 cup fresh raspberries

1/2 cup diced fresh tomatoes

1/2 cup Greek yogurt

1/4 cup almond milk

1/4 tsp vanilla extract

WATERMELON POMEGRANATE SMOOTHIE

1 cup watermelon chunks

1/2 cup pomegranate seeds

1/2 cup Greek yogurt

1/4 cup almond milk

1 tsp honey (optional)

RED BELL PEPPER BASIL SMOOTHIE

1/2 red bell pepper, diced

1/2 cup Greek yogurt

1/2 cup almond milk

1/4 cup fresh basil leaves

1 tsp honey (optional)

RED DRAGONFRUIT STRAWBERRY SMOOTHIE

1/2 cup fresh or frozen dragon fruit chunks

1/2 cup fresh or frozen strawberries

1/2 cup Greek yogurt

1/4 cup almond milk

1/4 tsp vanilla extract

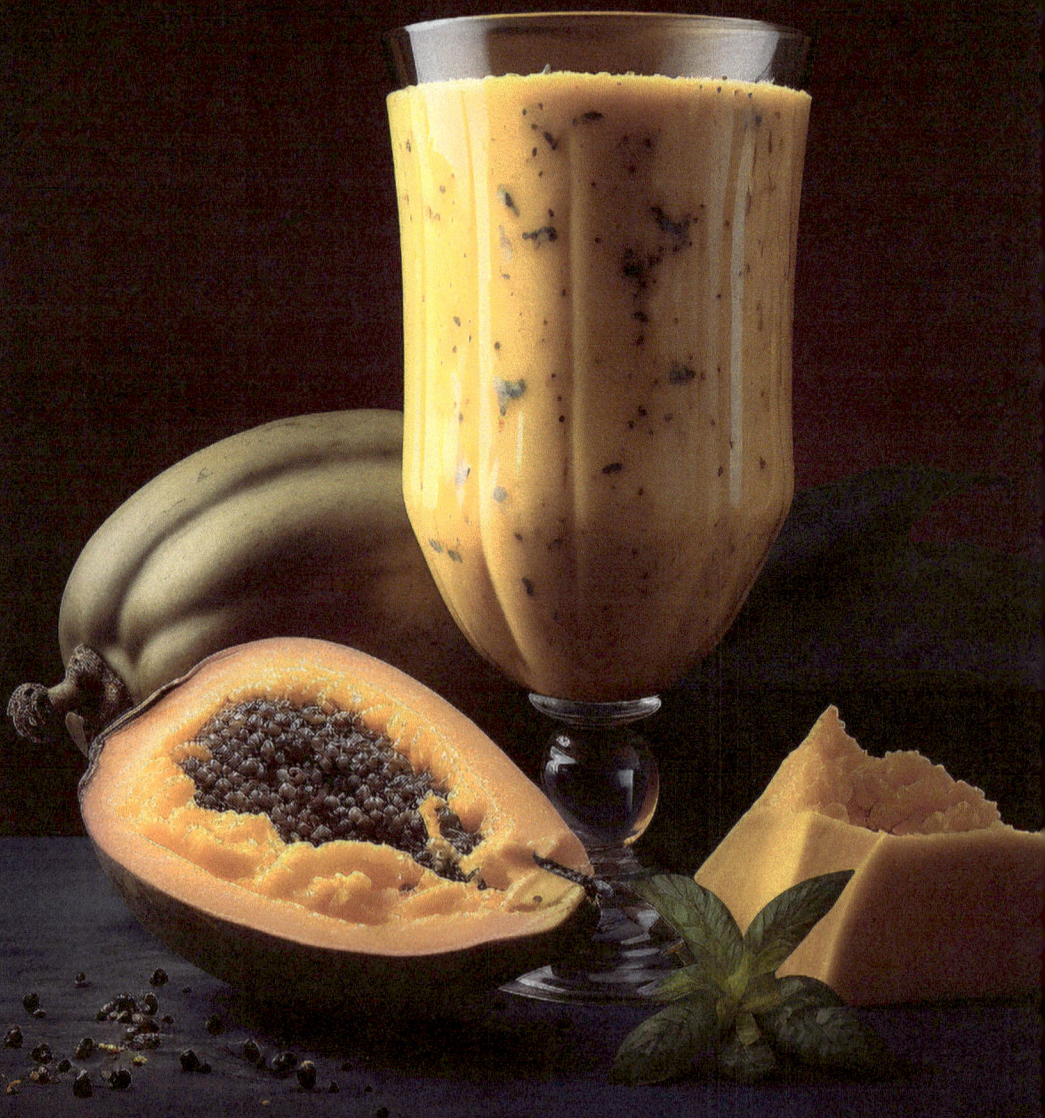

ORANGE PAPAYA
TURMERIC SMOOTHIE

CARROT ORANGE GINGER SMOOTHIE

1 cup diced carrots

1 orange, peeled and segmented

1/2 inch piece of ginger, peeled

1/2 cup Greek yogurt

1/2 cup orange juice

1 tsp honey (optional)

SWEET POTATO VANILLA SMOOTHIE

1/2 cup cooked and cooled sweet potato chunks

1/2 cup Greek yogurt

1/4 cup orange juice

1/4 tsp vanilla extract

1 tsp honey (optional)

ORANGE PAPAYA TURMERIC SMOOTHIE

1 orange, peeled and segmented

1/2 cup diced papaya

1/2 cup Greek yogurt

1/4 cup orange juice

1/4 tsp ground turmeric

APRICOT NECTARINE PAPRIKA SMOOTHIE

1 apricot, peeled and pitted

1 nectarine, peeled and pitted

1/2 cup Greek yogurt

1/4 cup orange juice

1/4 tsp paprika

1 tsp honey (optional)

ORANGE CANTALOUPE MARIGOLD SMOOTHIE

1 orange, peeled and segmented

1/2 cup diced cantaloupe

1/2 cup Greek yogurt

1/4 cup orange juice

2-3 marigold petals (or nasturtium)

As usual, ingredients amount can be adjusted to your preference. And honey is optional for sweetness, you can use any other sweetener you prefer or you can skip it if you like it less sweet.

Adding some orange-colored herbs such as marigold and nasturtium can give a unique taste to the smoothie, but it could be hard to find them fresh in certain location, so you can use dried petals or omit them if you can't find them.

Keep in mind that blending orange fruit with other ingredients also enhances the taste and also makes the smoothie more nutritious. You can also add some spices like ginger or cinnamon that are known for their anti-inflammatory properties and also add a subtle flavor to the smoothie.

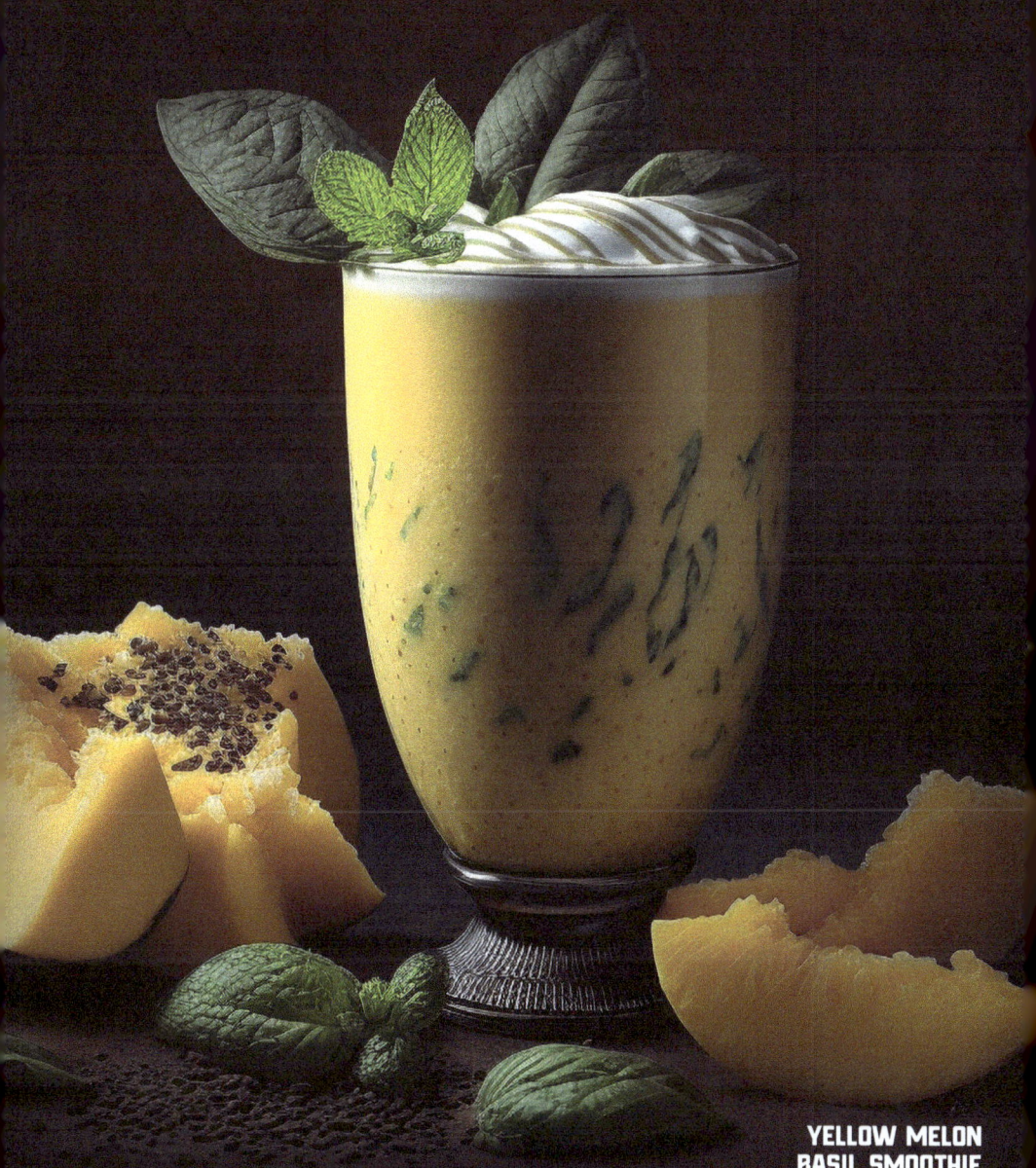

YELLOW MELON
BASIL SMOOTHIE

MANGO TURMERIC SMOOTHIE

1 ripe mango, peeled and diced

1/2 cup Greek yogurt

1/2 cup almond milk

1/2 tsp ground turmeric

1 tsp honey (optional)

LEMON GINGER SMOOTHIE

1 lemon, juiced

1/2 inch piece of ginger, peeled

1/2 cup Greek yogurt

1/2 cup almond milk

1 tsp honey (optional)

PINEAPPLE TURMERIC SMOOTHIE

1 cup pineapple chunks

1/2 cup Greek yogurt

1/4 cup almond milk

1/4 tsp vanilla extract

1/4 tsp ground turmeric

YELLOW SQUASH AND HONEY SMOOTHIE

1/2 cup cooked and cooled yellow squash chunks

1/2 cup Greek yogurt

1/4 cup almond milk

1 tsp honey

1/4 tsp vanilla extract

YELLOW MELON BASIL SMOOTHIE

1 cup diced yellow melon (cantaloupe or honeydew)

1/2 cup Greek yogurt

1/4 cup almond milk

1/4 tsp vanilla extract

1 handful of fresh basil leaves

BLUE / INDIGO
SMOOTHIES

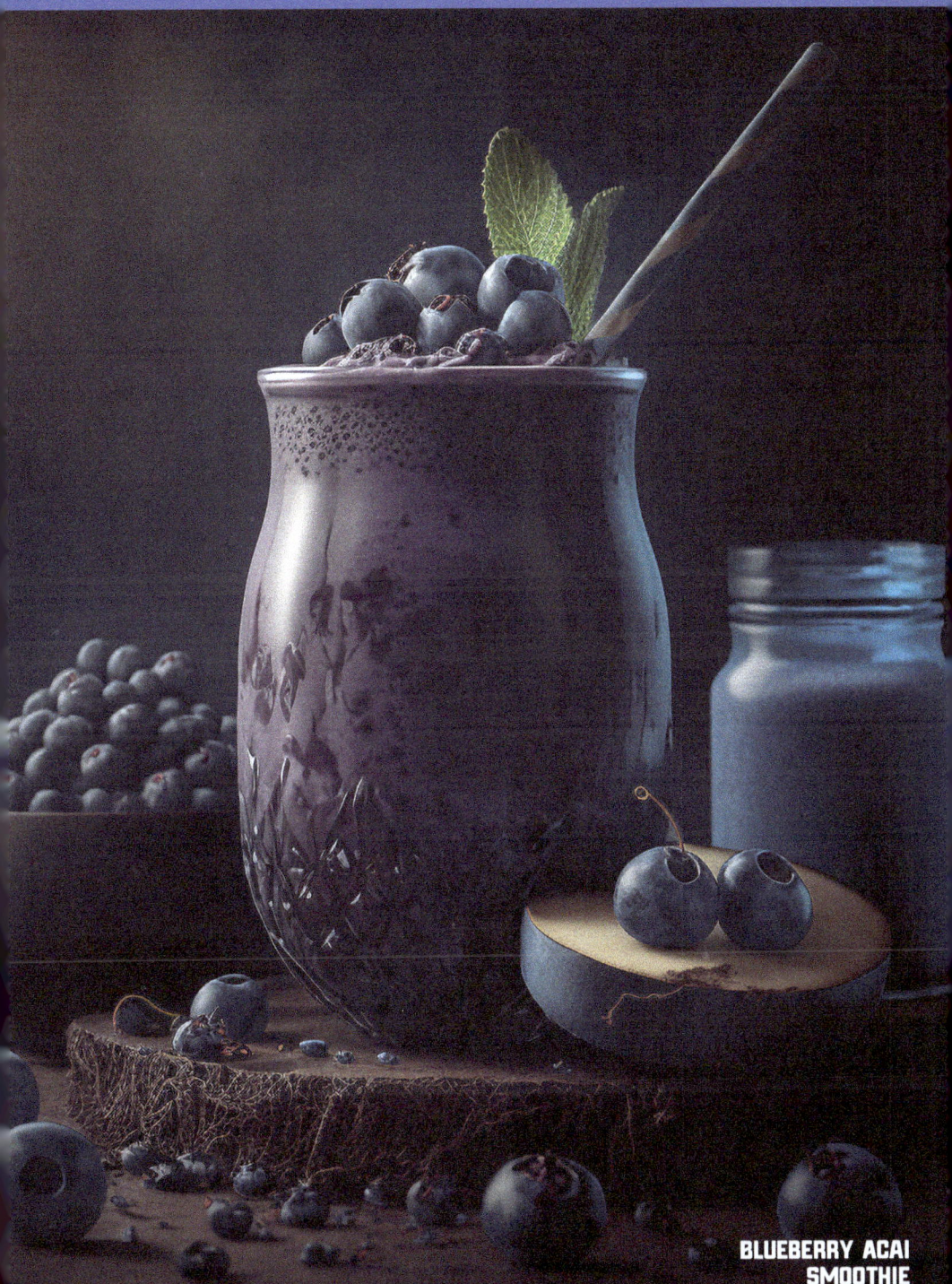

BLUEBERRY ACAI
SMOOTHIE

BLUEBERRY BLACKBERRY SMOOTHIE

1 cup fresh blueberries

1/2 cup fresh blackberries

1/2 cup Greek yogurt

1/4 cup almond milk

1 tsp honey (optional)

BLUE POTATO ELDERBERRY SMOOTHIE

1/2 cup cooked and cooled Blue Potato chunks

1/2 cup fresh or frozen elderberries

1/2 cup Greek yogurt

1/4 cup almond milk

1/4 tsp vanilla extract

BLUEBERRY BLACK CURRANT SMOOTHIE

1 cup fresh blueberries

1/2 cup fresh blackcurrants

1/2 cup Greek yogurt

1/4 cup almond milk

1/4 tsp vanilla extract

BLUEBERRY ACAI SMOOTHIE

1/2 cup frozen blueberries

1/2 cup frozen acai berries

1/2 cup Greek yogurt

1/4 cup almond milk

1 tsp honey (optional)

BLUE CORN SMOOTHIE

1/2 cup cooked and cooled blue corn kernels

1/2 cup Greek yogurt

1/4 cup almond milk

1/4 tsp vanilla extract

1 tsp honey (optional)

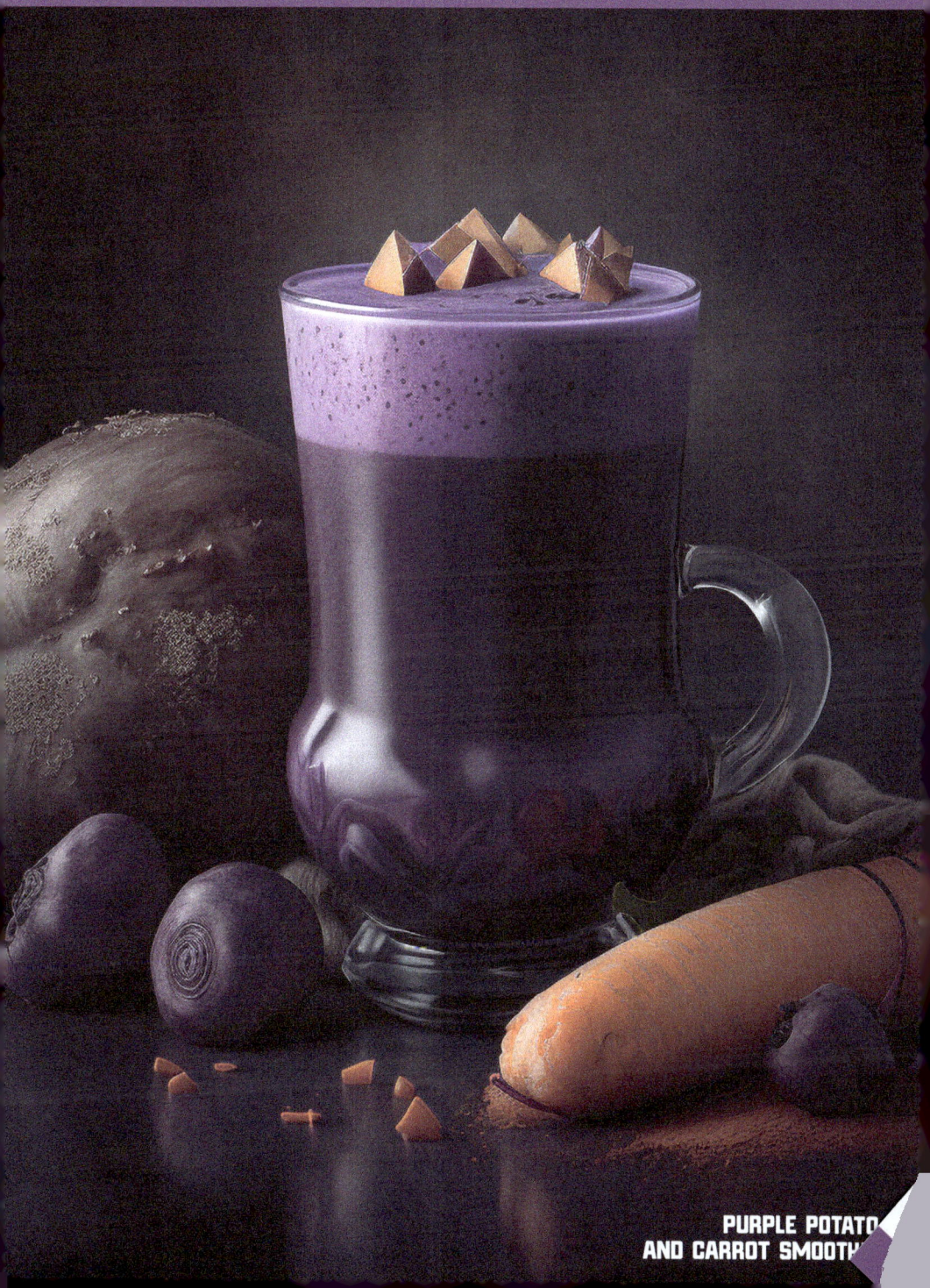

PURPLE / VIOLET
SMOOTHIES

PURPLE POTATO
AND CARROT SMOOTH...

BLUEBERRY BASIL BLISS

1 cup fresh blueberries

1 banana

1/2 cup fresh purple basil leaves

1/2 cup plain Greek yogurt

1 cup unsweetened almond milk

1 tsp honey (optional)

BLEND ALL INGREDIENTS TOGETHER UNTIL SMOOTH AND CREAMY

PLUMS AND PEACHES

1 cup fresh plums

1 peach

1/2 cup red grapes

1/4 cup plain Greek yogurt

1/2 cup unsweetened almond milk

1 tsp honey (optional)

BLEND ALL INGREDIENTS TOGETHER UNTIL SMOOTH AND CREAMY

BLACKBERRY BEET

1 cup fresh blackberries

1 small cooked beet

1/2 cup fresh purple basil leaves

1/2 cup plain Greek yogurt

1 cup unsweetened almond milk

1 tsp honey (optional)

BLEND ALL INGREDIENTS TOGETHER UNTIL SMOOTH AND CREAMY

PURPLE POTATO AND CARROT

1 small cooked purple potato

1 small cooked purple carrot

1/4 cup red grapes

1/2 cup unsweetened almond milk

1 tsp honey (optional)

BLEND ALL INGREDIENTS TOGETHER UNTIL SMOOTH AND CREAMY

EGGPLANT AND BLACK CURRANT

1/2 cup cooked eggplant

1/2 cup fresh black currants

1/2 cup plain Greek yogurt

1/2 cup unsweetened almond milk

1 tsp honey (optional)

BLEND ALL INGREDIENTS TOGETHER UNTIL SMOOTH AND CREAMY

BLACK
SMOOTHIES

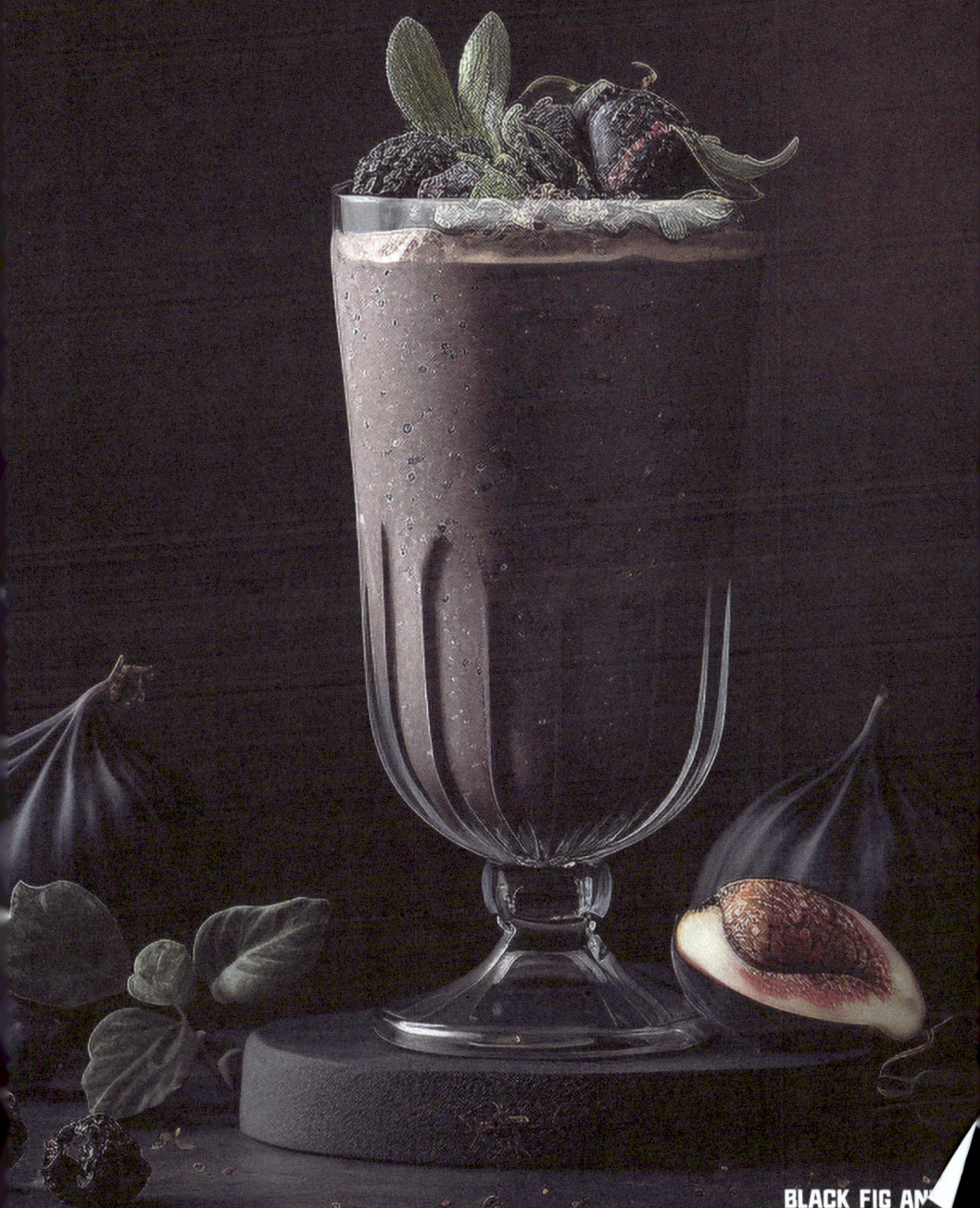

BLACK FIG AN
BLACK SAGE SMOOT

BLACKBERRY AND BLACK CURRANT SMOOTHIE

1 cup blackberries
1/2 cup black currants
1/2 banana
1/2 cup Greek yogurt
1/2 cup almond milk
1 tsp honey (optional)

BLEND ALL INGREDIENTS IN A BLENDER UNTIL SMOOTH

BLACK SESAME AND BLACK SOYBEAN SMOOTHIE

1/2 cup black soybeans (soaked overnight)
1 tbsp black sesame seeds
1/2 banana
1/2 cup Greek yogurt
1/2 cup almond milk
1 tsp honey (optional)

BLEND ALL INGREDIENTS IN A BLENDER UNTIL SMOOTH

BLACK NIGHTSHADE AND BLACK RADISH SMOOTHIE

1/2 cup black nightshade (cleaned and boiled)
* This is not deadly nightshade (Atropa belladonna)
1/4 cup sliced black radish
1/2 banana
1/2 cup Greek yogurt
1/2 cup almond milk
1 tsp honey (optional)

BLEND ALL INGREDIENTS IN A BLENDER UNTIL SMOOTH

BLACK ELDERBERRY AND BLACK GARLIC SMOOTHIE

1/2 cup black elderberries
2 cloves black garlic
1/2 banana
1/2 cup Greek yogurt
1/2 cup almond milk
1 tsp honey (optional)

BLEND ALL INGREDIENTS IN A BLENDER UNTIL SMOOTH

BLACK FIG AND BLACK SAGE SMOOTHIE

1/2 cup black figs
1 tsp dried black sage
1/2 banana
1/2 cup Greek yogurt
1/2 cup almond milk
1 tsp honey (optional)

BLEND ALL INGREDIENTS IN A BLENDER UNTIL SMOOTH

WHITE
SMOOTHIES

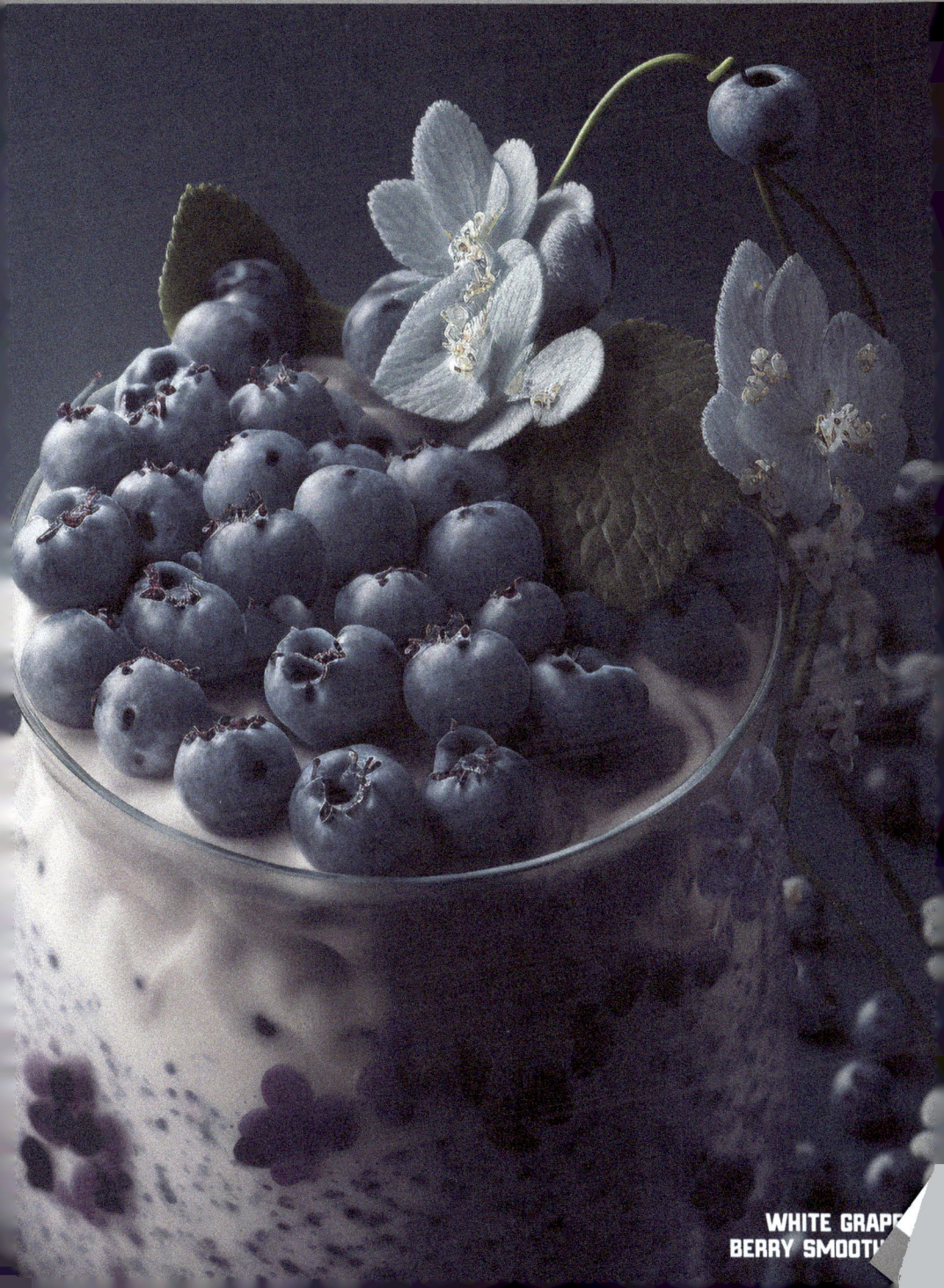

WHITE PEACH GINGER SMOOTHIE

1 white peach, peeled and pitted

1/2 cup coconut milk

1/2 cup Greek yogurt

1/2 inch piece of ginger, peeled

1/2 tsp honey (optional)

WHITE PEAR ROSEMARY SMOOTHIE

1 white pear, peeled and cored

1/2 cup Greek yogurt

1/2 cup coconut milk

1/2 tsp honey (optional)

1 sprig of rosemary

CAULIFLOWER PINEAPPLE SMOOTHIE

1/2 cup cooked and cooled cauliflower florets

1/2 cup pineapple chunks

1/2 cup coconut milk

1/4 cup Greek yogurt

1/4 tsp vanilla extract

WHITE NECTARINE BASIL SMOOTHIE

1 white nectarine, peeled and pitted

1/2 cup Greek yogurt

1/2 cup coconut milk

1/2 tsp honey (optional)

1 handful of fresh basil leaves

WHITE GRAPE BERRY SMOOTHIE

1 cup white grapes

1/2 cup blueberries

1/2 cup Greek yogurt

1/4 cup coconut milk

1/4 tsp vanilla extract

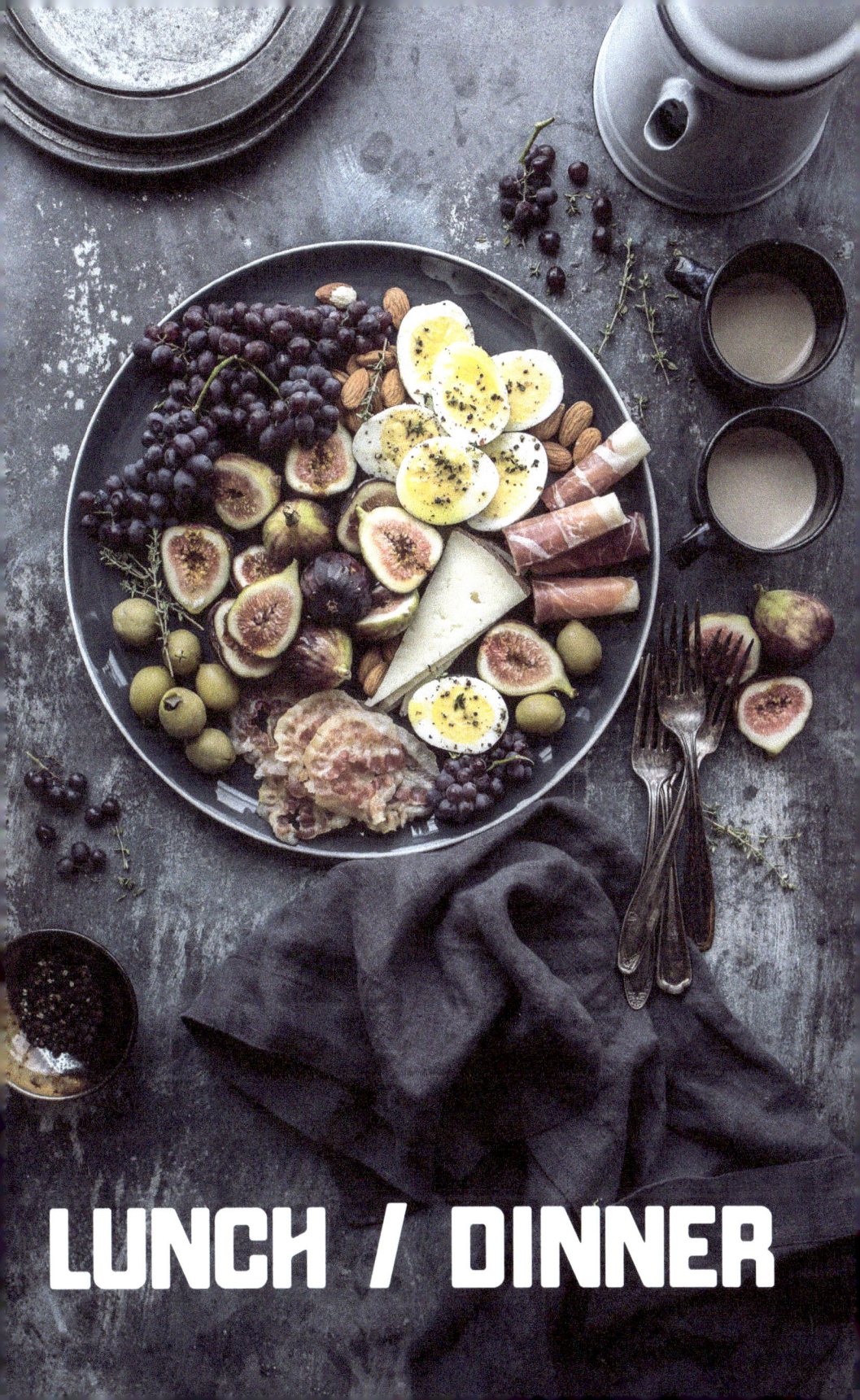

LUNCH / DINNER

Please note that this book does not necessarily promote vegetarianism or an omnivore (meat-eating) based diet.

In the following pages, I will give various examples of recipes with ingredients that can easily be substituted to better fit your diet.

For example, the cheese in most of these recipes could be eliminated, or the chicken could be replaced with a plant-based alternative such as lion's mane.

Many studies detail the dangers of consuming chemical-laden plant-based foods and foods with soy as an ingredient.

Be warned of these and many others hid under the 'Natural Flavors' labeling.

RED

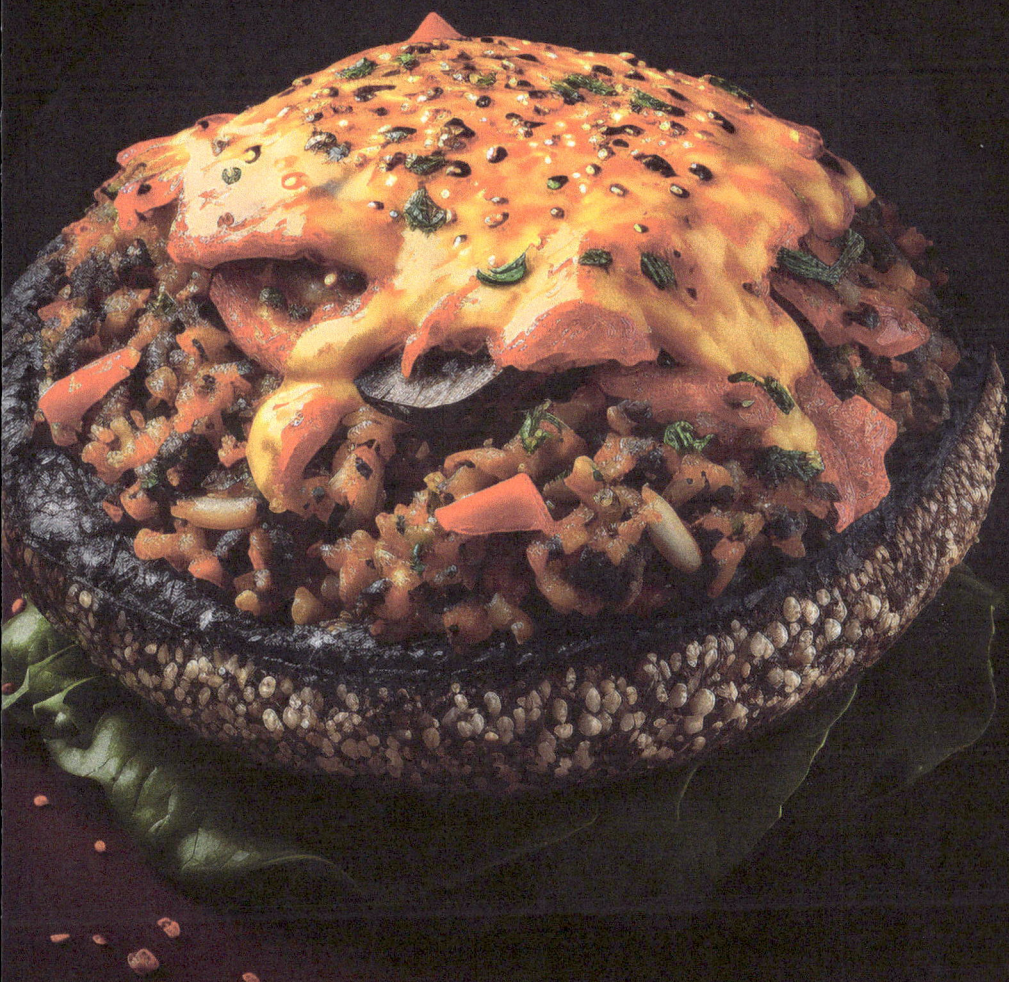

RED PEPPER AND LENTIL STUFFED PORTOBELLO MUSHROOMS

INGREDIENTS

4 large Portobello mushrooms, stems removed

1 cup of cooked lentils

2 red bell peppers, diced

1/4 cup of diced red onion

1 clove of garlic, minced

1/4 cup of chopped fresh parsley

1/4 cup of grated Parmesan cheese

2 tablespoons of olive oil

Salt and pepper to taste

DIRECTIONS

1. Preheat the oven to 375 degrees F.

2. Brush both sides of the mushrooms with 1 tablespoon of olive oil and season with salt and pepper.

3. In a pan over medium heat, sauté the red bell peppers, red onion, and garlic in the remaining olive oil until they are tender.

4. Add the cooked lentils and sauté for 2-3 minutes more.

5. Remove the pan from the heat and stir in the parsley and Parmesan cheese.

6. Stuff each mushroom with the lentil mixture, mounding it slightly on top.

7. Place the mushrooms on a baking sheet and bake for 15-20 minutes, or until the mushrooms are tender and the filling is heated through.

8. Remove from the oven and let them cool for a few minutes.

9. Serve them as a main course or side dish.

This recipe is a delicious and healthy way to enjoy red-skinned vegetables, in this case red bell pepper, as the star ingredient. The portobello mushrooms make a great meaty base for the lentil mixture, and the Parmesan cheese adds a nice richness and flavor. This recipe is also a good source of protein and fiber. As always, make sure to adjust seasoning and ingredients according to personal preference, dietary restrictions or ingredient availability.

RED CURRY WITH RED VEGETABLES

INGREDIENTS

1 tablespoon of coconut oil

2 cloves of garlic, minced

1 tablespoon of red curry paste

1 red bell pepper, sliced

1 red onion, sliced

1 cup of cherry tomatoes, halved

1 cup of diced red potatoes

1 can of coconut milk

1/4 cup of chopped fresh basil

1/4 cup of chopped fresh cilantro

Salt and pepper to taste

Cooked jasmine rice for serving

DIRECTIONS

1. Heat the coconut oil in a large pan over medium heat.

2. Add the garlic and curry paste and sauté for 1-2 minutes until fragrant.

3. Add the red bell pepper, red onion, cherry tomatoes, and diced red potatoes. Sauté for 5-7 minutes, or until the vegetables are tender.

4. Pour in the coconut milk and bring the mixture to a simmer.

5. Reduce the heat to low and let the curry simmer for 10-15 minutes.

6. Season with salt and pepper to taste.

7. Stir in the basil and cilantro and cook for 1 more minute.

8. Serve the curry over cooked jasmine rice and enjoy!

This recipe is a flavorful and hearty dish that highlights red vegetables as the main ingredient, in this case red bell pepper, cherry tomatoes and red onion. The red curry paste and coconut milk give it a rich and creamy sauce. This recipe is also vegan-friendly and gluten-free. The jasmine rice helps to balance the spice and the herbs provide a nice freshness. As always, make sure to adjust seasoning and ingredients according to personal preference, dietary restrictions or ingredient availability.

RED PEPPER AND TOMATO RISOTTO

INGREDIENTS

1 tablespoon of olive oil

1 red onion, diced

2 red bell peppers, diced

2 cloves of garlic, minced

2 cups of cherry tomatoes, halved

1 cup of Arborio rice

3 cups of vegetable broth

1/4 cup of grated Parmesan cheese

1/4 cup of chopped fresh basil

Salt and pepper to taste

DIRECTIONS

1. Heat the olive oil in a large pan over medium heat.

2. Add the red onion, red bell peppers, and garlic and sauté for 5-7 minutes, or until the vegetables are tender.

3. Add the cherry tomatoes and sauté for an additional 2-3 minutes.

4. Stir in the Arborio rice and cook for 1-2 minutes, until the rice is lightly toasted.

5. Gradually add the vegetable broth, stirring constantly. Bring the mixture to a simmer and reduce the heat to low.

6. Cook the risotto, stirring frequently, for 18-20 minutes, or until the rice is tender and the risotto is creamy.

7. Remove the pan from the heat and stir in the grated Parmesan cheese, chopped basil, salt and pepper.

8. Serve the risotto in bowls and enjoy!

This recipe is a delicious and comforting dish that features red bell peppers, cherry tomatoes and red onion as the main ingredient. Arborio rice and parmesan cheese give it a creamy texture, while the basil adds a fresh, herby flavor. This recipe is also a good source of fiber, protein, and antioxidants. This dish can be served as a main course or side dish. As always, make sure to adjust seasoning and ingredients according to personal preference, dietary restrictions or ingredient availability.

ORANGE

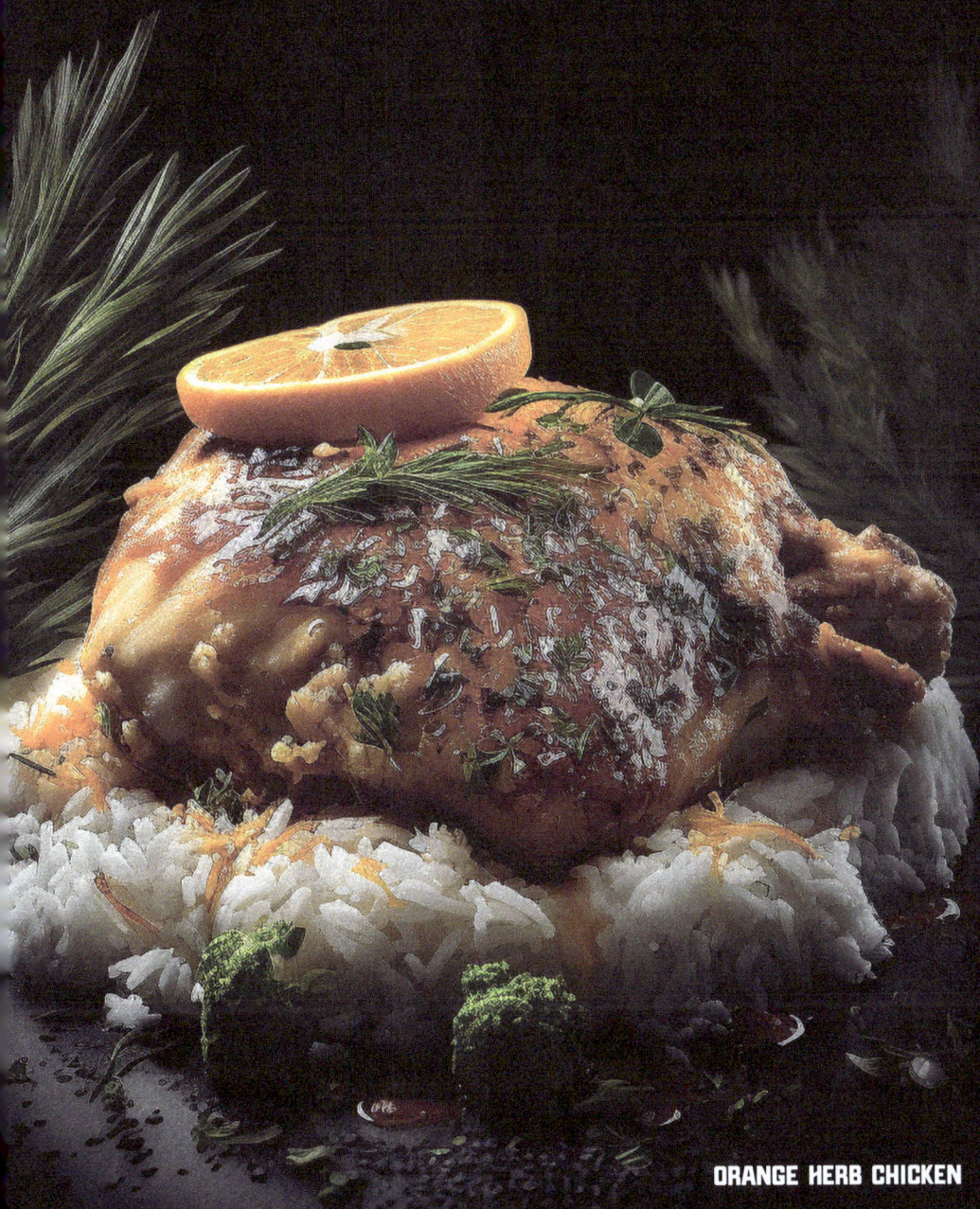

ORANGE HERB CHICKEN

ORANGE HERB SALAD

INGREDIENTS

2 oranges, peeled
and segmented

1 grapefruit, peeled
and segmented

1 medium-sized
sweet potato,
peeled and diced

1 medium-sized
red onion,
thinly sliced

1/4 cup chopped
fresh parsley

1/4 cup chopped
fresh basil

2 tbsp olive oil

1 tbsp honey

Salt and pepper
to taste

DIRECTIONS

1. Preheat the oven to 375 degrees F.

2. Toss the diced sweet potato
   in 1 tbsp of olive oil and season
   with salt and pepper. Spread out
   on a baking sheet and roast for
   20-25 minutes, or until tender
   and lightly browned.

3. In a small bowl, whisk together
   the remaining 1 tbsp of olive oil
   and honey. Season with salt
   and pepper to taste.

4. In a large bowl, combine the orange
   segments, grapefruit segments, roasted
   sweet potato, and sliced red onion.

5. Drizzle the honey and olive oil mixture
   over the salad and toss to coat.

6. Sprinkle the chopped parsley
   and basil over the top of the salad
   and toss to combine.

7. Serve immediately, and Enjoy your
   delicious and healthy dinner!

Note: you can add some nuts, seeds or even some cheese if you want to
make it more filling.

ORANGE HERB RISOTTO

INGREDIENTS

1 cup Arborio rice

2 cups chicken or vegetable broth

1/2 cup dry white wine

1/2 cup grated Parmesan cheese

1 tbsp olive oil

1 small onion, finely diced

2 cloves of garlic, minced

1 orange, zest and juice

1 medium-sized carrot, peeled and grated

1/4 cup chopped fresh thyme

Salt and pepper to taste

DIRECTIONS

1. In a medium-sized saucepan, bring the chicken or vegetable broth to a simmer and keep it warm over low heat.

2. In a large heavy-bottomed pot or Dutch oven, heat the olive oil over medium heat. Add the onion and garlic and cook until softened, about 5 minutes.

3. Add the Arborio rice and stir to coat with the oil. Cook for 1-2 minutes or until the rice is lightly toasted.

4. Add the white wine and stir until the liquid is absorbed.

5. Begin adding the hot broth to the rice mixture, about 1/2 cup at a time, stirring constantly until each addition is absorbed before adding the next.

6. Once the rice is cooked through, and the mixture creamy and tender, remove from the heat and stir in the grated Parmesan cheese, grated carrot, orange zest, orange juice, chopped thyme and season with salt and pepper to taste.

7. Serve the risotto in bowls and garnish with more Parmesan cheese and fresh thyme if desired.

8. Enjoy your delicious and healthy dinner!

Note: you can add some shrimp or chicken if you want to make it more protein rich.

ORANGE HERB CHICKEN

INGREDIENTS

4 boneless, skinless chicken breasts

1/4 cup flour

Salt and pepper

2 tbsp olive oil

2 cloves of garlic, minced

1/4 cup orange juice

1 tbsp honey

1 tbsp grainy mustard

1/4 tsp smoked paprika

1 medium-sized red bell pepper, seeded and sliced

1 medium-sized yellow onion, sliced

2 medium-sized carrots, peeled and sliced

1/4 cup chopped fresh thyme

1/4 cup chopped fresh parsley

DIRECTIONS

1. Preheat oven to 375 degrees F (190 degrees C). Grease a baking dish.

2. Season chicken with flour, salt, and pepper. In a large skillet, heat olive oil over medium-high heat. Add chicken and cook until browned on both sides, about 3 minutes per side. Remove chicken from skillet and place in the prepared baking dish.

3. In the same skillet, add garlic, orange juice, honey, mustard, and smoked paprika. Stir to combine and bring to a simmer.

4. Add the sliced bell pepper, onion, and carrot to the skillet and stir to coat with the sauce.

5. Pour the mixture over the chicken in the baking dish. Sprinkle with thyme and parsley.

6. Bake in the preheated oven for 25-30 minutes, or until the chicken is cooked through.

7. Serve and enjoy your delicious and healthy dinner!

Note: You can also add some potatoes or another grain to make it a complete meal.

YELLOW

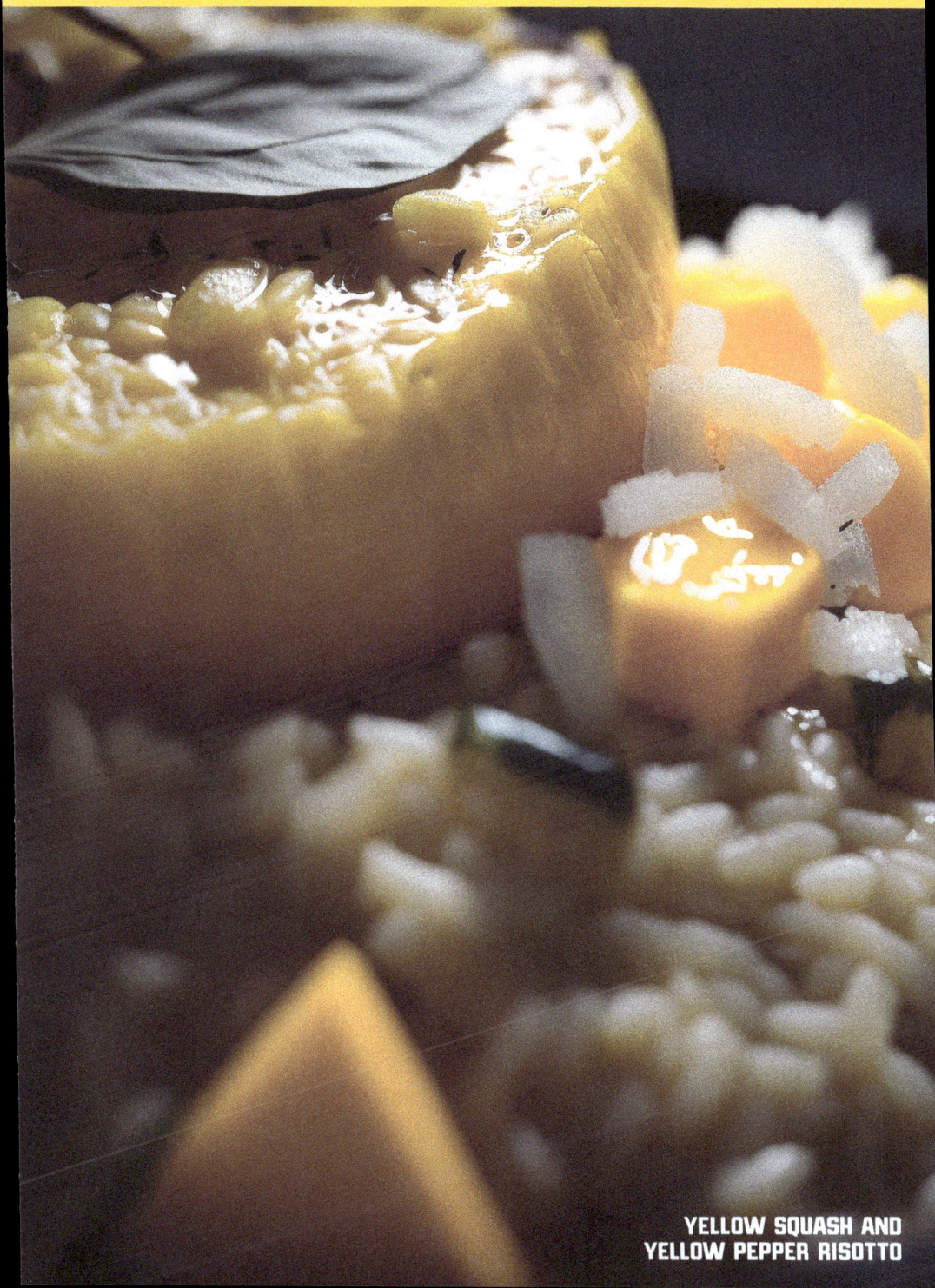

YELLOW SQUASH AND
YELLOW PEPPER RISOTTO

ELLOW SQUASH AND YELLOW PEPPER RISOTTO

INGREDIENTS

1 yellow onion, diced

3 cloves of garlic, minced

2 yellow bell peppers, diced

2 yellow squash, diced

1 cup of Arborio rice

1/2 cup of white wine

4 cups of vegetable or chicken stock

1/4 cup of grated Parmesan cheese

2 tablespoons of chopped fresh basil

2 tablespoons of chopped fresh thyme

Salt and pepper, to taste

Olive oil, for cooking

DIRECTIONS

1. Heat a large skillet over medium heat and add olive oil.

2. Add the diced onion and garlic and sauté until softened, about 5 minutes.

3. Add the diced yellow bell peppers and yellow squash to the skillet and sauté for another 5 minutes.

4. Stir in the Arborio rice and cook for 2 minutes to coat the rice with the vegetables and oil.

5. Pour in the white wine and stir until it has been absorbed by the rice.

6. Slowly pour in the stock, one cup at a time, stirring constantly until each cup has been absorbed before adding the next.

7. Continue cooking and stirring until the risotto is creamy and the rice is cooked through, about 20 minutes.

8. Remove the skillet from heat and stir in the grated Parmesan cheese, chopped basil and thyme.

9. Season with salt and pepper to taste.

10. Serve the risotto hot and garnish with additional fresh basil and thyme, if desired.

Enjoy the bright and delicious combination of yellow skinned fruits and vegetables in this creamy risotto dish. The yellow bell peppers and yellow squash add a nice sweetness and texture to the dish, while the herbs and Parmesan cheese give it a nice depth of flavor. This dish is a perfect main course for a summer dinner party.

YELLOW CURRY CHICKEN WITH YELLOW POTATOES AND YELLOW TOMATOES

INGREDIENTS

2 lb boneless, skinless chicken thighs, cut into bite-size pieces

2 yellow potatoes, peeled and diced

2 yellow tomatoes, diced

1 yellow onion, diced

2 cloves of garlic, minced

1 tablespoon of yellow curry powder

1 teaspoon of ground turmeric

1/2 teaspoon of ground cumin

1/4 teaspoon of ground cinnamon

1 can of coconut milk

2 cups of chicken broth

2 tablespoons of fish sauce

1 tablespoon of brown sugar

2 tablespoons of fresh cilantro, chopped

2 tablespoons of fresh basil, chopped

Salt and pepper, to taste

Cooking oil, for cooking

DIRECTIONS

1. Heat a large pot over medium-high heat and add cooking oil.

2. Add the chicken pieces and cook until browned on all sides, about 5 minutes.

3. Remove the chicken from the pot and set aside.

4. In the same pot, add more oil if needed and sauté the diced onions and garlic until softened, about 5 minutes.

5. Add the diced yellow potatoes, yellow tomatoes, curry powder, turmeric, cumin, and cinnamon. Cook for 2-3 minutes or until fragrant.

6. Add the chicken back to the pot along with the coconut milk, chicken broth, fish sauce, and brown sugar.

7. Bring the curry to a simmer and let it cook for about 20 minutes or until the chicken and potatoes are cooked through and the curry has thickened.

8. Stir in the chopped cilantro and basil. Season with salt and pepper to taste.

9. Serve the curry over steamed jasmine rice and garnish with additional cilantro and basil.

This yellow curry dish is packed with flavor and nutrition. The yellow curry powder, turmeric and cumin gives it a delicious and aromatic taste while the yellow potatoes and yellow tomatoes gives it a nice texture and sweetness. The chicken thighs, coconut milk and chicken broth gives it a rich and creamy base. The fresh herbs and fish sauce gives it a fresh and savory touch. This dish is a perfect main course for a hearty dinner.

YELLOW SUMMER VEGETABLE TART

INGREDIENTS

1 pre-made pie crust

2 yellow summer squash, sliced

2 yellow bell peppers, sliced

1 yellow onion, sliced

2 cloves of garlic, minced

2 tablespoons of olive oil

Salt and pepper, to taste

3 eggs

1/2 cup of heavy cream

1/2 cup of grated Parmesan cheese

1/4 cup of chopped fresh thyme

1/4 cup of chopped fresh basil

DIRECTIONS

1. Preheat the oven to 375°F (190°C).

2. Roll out the pie crust and press it into a 9-inch tart pan. Prick the bottom of the crust with a fork.

3. In a large skillet over medium heat, add olive oil. Add the sliced yellow summer squash, yellow bell peppers, yellow onion, and garlic. Cook until the vegetables are soft and lightly browned, about 10 minutes. Season with salt and pepper to taste.

4. In a mixing bowl, whisk together the eggs, heavy cream, grated Parmesan cheese, thyme, and basil. Season with salt and pepper to taste.

5. Spread the cooked vegetables over the pie crust. Pour the egg mixture over the vegetables.

6. Bake the tart for 25-30 minutes or until the crust is golden brown and the filling is set.

7. Let the tart cool for a few minutes before slicing and serving.

This savory vegetable tart is perfect for a summer dinner party. The yellow summer squash and yellow bell peppers give the dish a bright pop of color and a nice sweetness, while the thyme and basil give it a nice depth of flavor. The eggs and cream give it a rich and creamy texture while the parmesan cheese add a nice nutty flavor. This dish is easy to make and delicious, it's a great way to use the yellow skinned fruits and vegetables that are in season during the summer.

GREEN

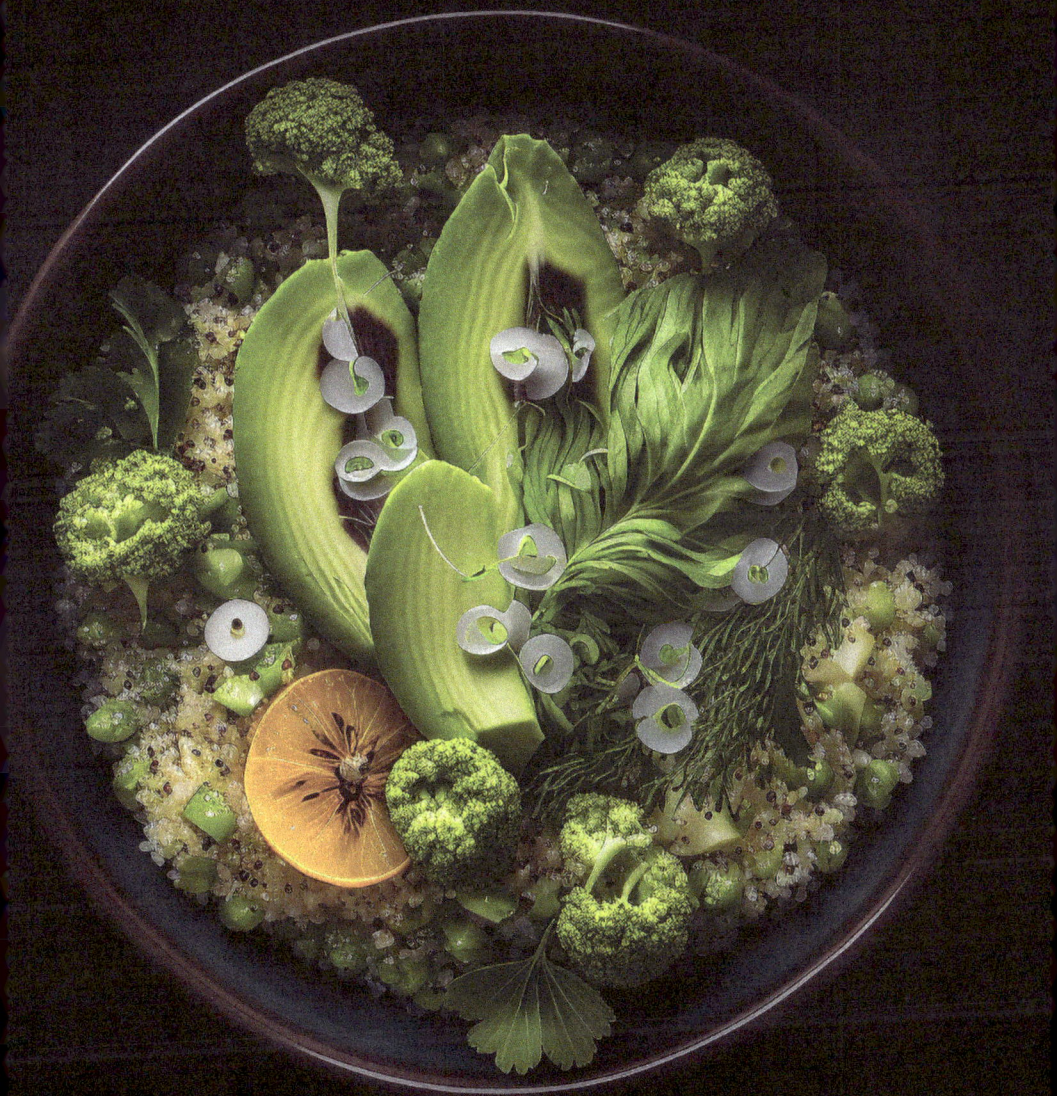

GREEN FRUIT, VEGETABLE
AND HERB QUINOA BOWL

GREEN HERB SALAD WITH GRILLED CHICKEN

INGREDIENTS

4 boneless, skinless chicken breasts

1/4 cup olive oil

2 tbsp lemon juice

1 tsp honey

1 tsp Dijon mustard

1/2 tsp dried thyme

Salt and pepper

2 avocados, diced

1 kiwi, peeled and diced

1 green apple, diced

1/2 cup green grapes, halved

1/4 cup chopped fresh mint

1/4 cup chopped fresh parsley

2 tbsp chopped fresh chives

2 tbsp chopped fresh basil

DIRECTIONS

1. In a small bowl, whisk together olive oil, lemon juice, honey, Dijon mustard, thyme, and a pinch of salt and pepper.

2. Place chicken in a large resealable bag, and pour marinade over the chicken. Seal the bag and toss to coat chicken evenly. Marinate for at least 30 minutes or up to 2 hours.

3. Preheat grill to medium-high heat. Grill chicken for about 6 minutes per side, or until cooked through.

4. In a large bowl, combine diced avocados, kiwi, green apple, grapes, mint, parsley, chives and basil.

5. Once chicken is done, let it cool for a few minutes and then slice them.

6. Add the sliced chicken to the bowl with the fruits and vegetables, and toss to combine.

7. Serve the salad in individual bowls and enjoy!

This is a light, refreshing salad with a perfect combination of sweet and savory flavors, it's perfect for a summer dinner or a healthy lunch.

GREEN FRUIT, VEGETABLE AND HERB QUINOA BOWL

INGREDIENTS

1 cup quinoa

2 cups vegetable broth

1 tbsp olive oil

1 small zucchini, diced

1 small avocado, diced

1 kiwi, peeled and diced

1 green apple, diced

1/4 cup chopped fresh mint

1/4 cup chopped fresh parsley

2 tbsp chopped fresh chives

2 tbsp chopped fresh basil

2 tbsp lemon juice

Salt and pepper to taste

DIRECTIONS

1. Rinse quinoa in a fine-mesh strainer under cold running water for a minute.

2. In a medium saucepan, combine the quinoa, vegetable broth, and a pinch of salt. Bring to a boil, then reduce heat to low, cover and simmer for about 20 minutes or until quinoa is cooked through and tender.

3. Remove from heat and let it sit for 5 minutes. Fluff quinoa with a fork and transfer to a large bowl.

4. In a large skillet over medium-high heat, heat olive oil. Add diced zucchini, cook until tender, around 5 minutes.

5. Remove skillet from heat and let cool for a few minutes.

6. Add diced avocado, kiwi, green apple, mint, parsley, chives, basil and lemon juice to the skillet and stir to combine.

7. Add the skillet mixture to the bowl with the quinoa and toss to combine. Season with salt and pepper to taste.

8. Serve the quinoa bowl in individual bowls and enjoy!

This is a healthy, flavorful and filling dinner option, it's a great way to include a variety of green skinned fruits and vegetables in one dish. The quinoa provides a good source of plant-based protein, and the combination of herbs and lemon juice give a fresh and unique flavor to the dish. You can top it with your favorite sauce or dressing for extra flavor.

GREEN VEGETABLE AND HERB PASTA

INGREDIENTS

1 pound of spaghetti or your favorite pasta

1 tbsp olive oil

2 cloves of garlic, minced

1 small broccoli florets

1 small zucchini, diced

1/2 cup peas

1/2 cup diced green apples

1/4 cup chopped fresh mint

1/4 cup chopped fresh parsley

2 tbsp chopped fresh chives

2 tbsp chopped fresh basil

1/4 cup grated Parmesan cheese

Salt and pepper to taste

DIRECTIONS

1. Cook pasta in a large pot of salted water according to package instructions until al dente.

2. Reserve 1 cup of pasta cooking water and drain the pasta.

3. In a large skillet, heat olive oil over medium heat. Add garlic and sauté for 1 minute.

4. Add broccoli florets, zucchini and peas. Cook for 5-7 minutes or until tender.

5. Add diced green apples, mint, parsley, chives, basil, and a pinch of salt and pepper. Cook for another 1-2 minutes.

6. Add the cooked pasta and 1/2 cup of pasta cooking water to the skillet and toss to combine. Cook for 1-2 minutes or until pasta is heated through.

7. Remove skillet from heat and stir in grated Parmesan cheese.

8. Serve the pasta in individual bowls and enjoy!

This is a delicious and hearty dinner option that combines a variety of green skinned fruits, vegetables and herbs to give a unique and flavorful taste. The pasta and vegetables are coated in a light and herbaceous sauce that is made from the combination of herbs and Parmesan cheese. You can add some protein, such as grilled chicken or shrimp to make it more filling and satisfying.

BLUE / INDIGO

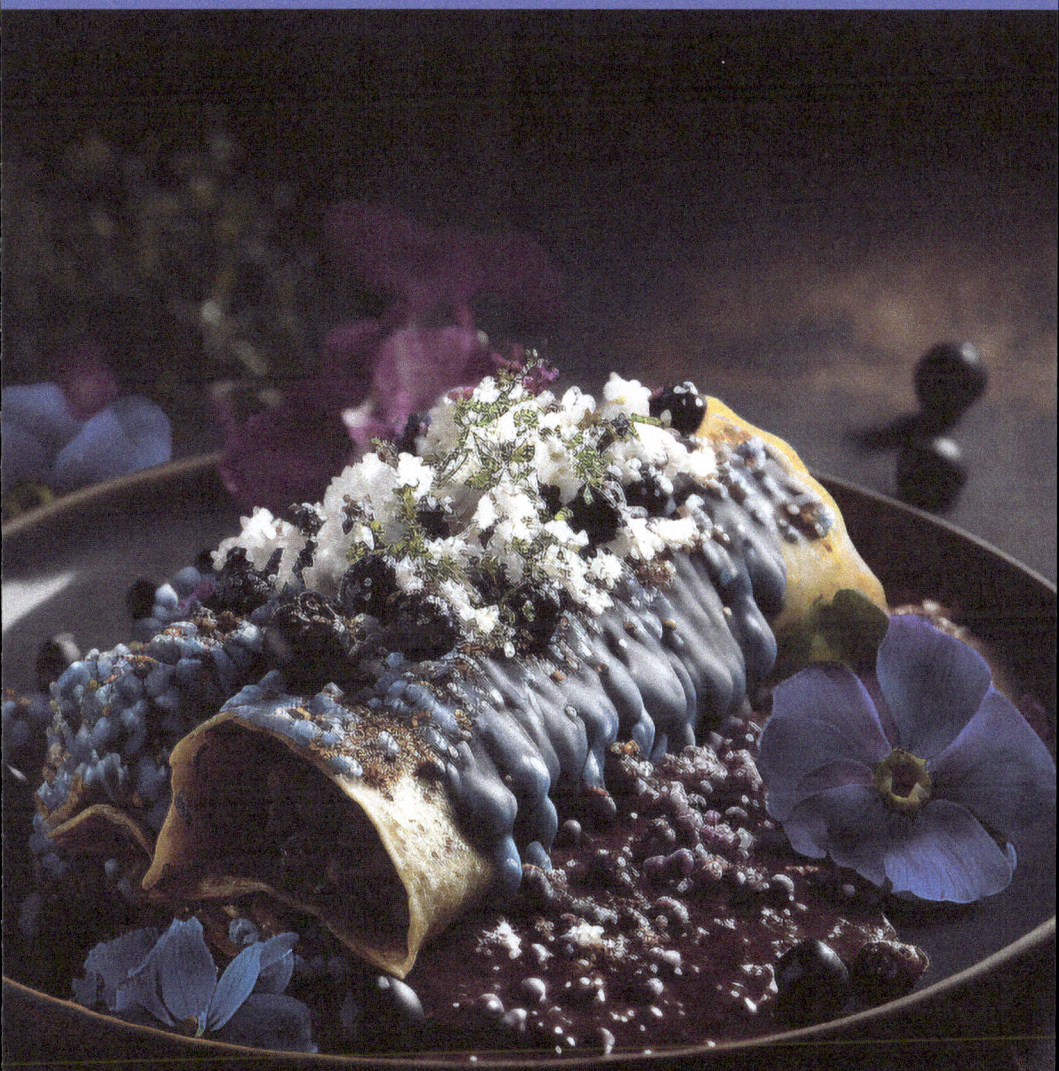

BLUEBERRY AND BLACKBERRY GRILLED CHICKEN SALAD

INGREDIENTS

2 boneless, skinless chicken breasts

1/4 cup fresh blueberries

1/4 cup fresh blackberries

2 tbsp olive oil

1 tsp dried thyme

1/2 tsp salt

1/4 tsp black pepper

1/4 cup red onion, thinly sliced

1/4 cup crumbled feta cheese

1/4 cup chopped fresh basil

2 tbsp balsamic vinegar

1 tbsp honey

DIRECTIONS

1. Preheat the grill to medium-high heat.

2. In a small bowl, combine the blueberries, blackberries, 1 tablespoon of olive oil, thyme, salt, and pepper. Mix well.

3. Place the chicken on the grill and brush with the berry mixture. Grill for 6-8 minutes per side, or until the chicken is cooked through.

4. Remove the chicken from the grill and let it rest for 5 minutes.

5. In a large bowl, combine the red onion, feta cheese, basil, balsamic vinegar, honey, and remaining 1 tablespoon of olive oil.

6. Slice the chicken and add it to the bowl. Toss to coat the chicken with the dressing.

7. Serve the chicken salad on a bed of mixed greens or with grilled bread. Enjoy!

You may also add some indigo-skinned fruits like blue potatoes, purple carrots or indigo basil to your salad to make it more colorful and delicious.

BLUE CORN ENCHILADAS WITH BLUEBERRY SALSA

INGREDIENTS

8 corn tortillas

1 cup cooked
blue corn kernels

1 cup cooked
black beans

1/2 cup crumbled
queso fresco

1/4 cup chopped
fresh cilantro

1/4 cup chopped
red onion

1/4 cup chopped
fresh blueberries

1/4 cup chopped
fresh blackberries

2 tbsp lime juice

2 tbsp honey

1 tsp ground cumin

1 tsp chili powder

Salt and pepper
to taste

1 cup enchilada sauce

DIRECTIONS

1. Preheat the oven to 375 degrees F.

2. In a mixing bowl, combine the blue corn kernels, black beans, queso fresco, cilantro, red onion, cumin, chili powder, salt and pepper. Mix well.

3. Spread about 1/4 cup of the enchilada sauce in the bottom of a baking dish.

4. Place a tortilla on a flat surface, and spoon about 2 tablespoons of the corn mixture onto the center of the tortilla. Roll the tortilla around the filling and place it seam-side down in the baking dish. Repeat with the remaining tortillas and filling.

5. Pour the remaining enchilada sauce over the top of the enchiladas.

6. In a small bowl, combine the blueberries, blackberries, lime juice, honey, and a pinch of salt. Mix well.

7. Spread the blueberry salsa over the top of the enchiladas.

8. Bake for 25-30 minutes, or until the enchiladas are heated through and the sauce is bubbly.

9. Serve the enchiladas with a side of purple cabbage and indigo basil, Enjoy!

BLUE POTATO GNOCCHI WITH BLUEBERRY SAGE BUTTER

INGREDIENTS

2 cups blue potatoes, peeled and diced

1 cup all-purpose flour

1 egg

1 tsp salt

1/4 cup fresh blueberries

2 tbsp butter

2 tbsp chopped fresh sage

1/4 cup grated Parmesan cheese

Salt and pepper to taste

DIRECTIONS

1. Boil the blue potatoes in a pot of salted water until tender, about 15-20 minutes. Drain and mash the potatoes until smooth.

2. In a large mixing bowl, combine the mashed potatoes, flour, egg, and salt. Mix until a dough forms.

3. On a lightly floured surface, roll the dough into long ropes, about 1/2 inch thick. Cut the ropes into small, 1-inch long gnocchi.

4. Bring a pot of salted water to a boil. Gently add the gnocchi to the water and cook for 2-3 minutes, or until they float to the surface.

5. In a small saucepan, melt the butter over medium heat. Add the blueberries and sage. Cook for 2-3 minutes, or until the blueberries start to burst.

6. Drain the gnocchi and add them to the saucepan with the butter sauce. Toss to coat the gnocchi evenly.

7. Serve the gnocchi in bowls, and top with grated Parmesan cheese, salt and pepper to taste. Enjoy!

You can garnish with fresh indigo basil or purple basil for extra aesthetic.

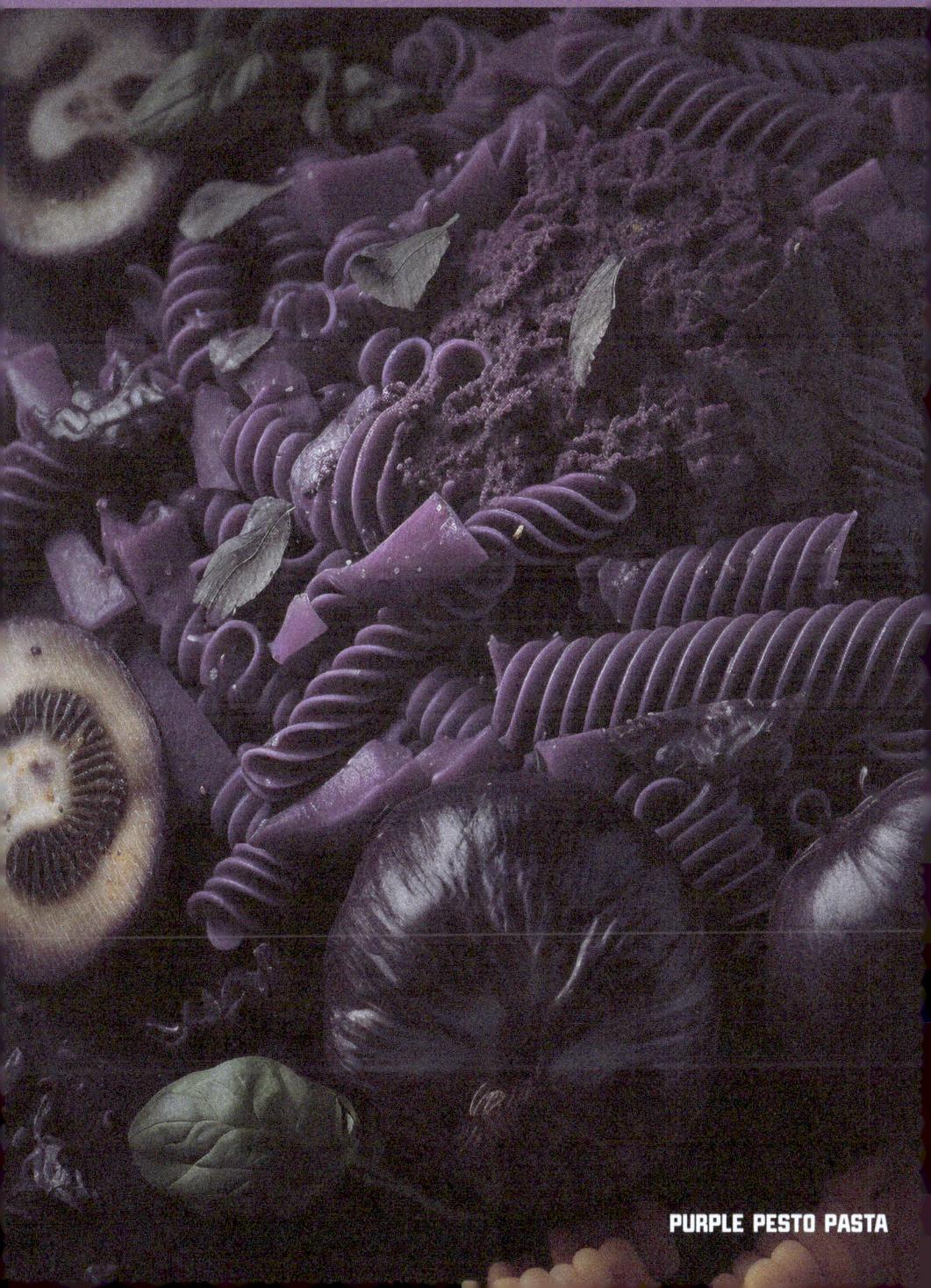

PURPLE / VIOLET

PURPLE PESTO PASTA

PURPLE VEGETABLE PAELLA

INGREDIENTS

1 cup Arborio rice

1 medium purple onion, diced

2 cloves of garlic, minced

1 red bell pepper, diced

1 cup purple grapes, halved

1 cup purple cauliflower florets

1 cup purple carrots, sliced

1/2 cup purple potatoes, diced

1/2 cup purple cherry tomatoes, halved

1 teaspoon smoked paprika

1 teaspoon dried thyme

1/2 teaspoon saffron threads

1/4 cup fresh parsley, chopped

3 cups vegetable broth

2 tablespoons olive oil

Salt and pepper, to taste

DIRECTIONS

1. Heat the olive oil in a large paella pan or skillet over medium heat.

2. Add the onions and garlic, sauté for 3-4 minutes or until softened.

3. Stir in the red bell pepper, purple grapes, purple cauliflower, purple carrots, purple potatoes, and cherry tomatoes. Cook for 5-7 minutes or until the vegetables are slightly tender.

4. Stir in the smoked paprika, thyme, saffron, and fresh parsley. Cook for 1-2 minutes or until fragrant.

5. Add the rice and stir to coat in the vegetables and spices. Cook for 1-2 minutes or until the rice is translucent.

6. Pour in the vegetable broth, bring the mixture to a simmer, and reduce the heat to low.

7. Cover the pan and cook for 18-20 minutes or until the rice is cooked through and the liquid has been absorbed.

8. Fluff the rice with a fork and season with salt and pepper to taste.

9. Serve hot and garnish with additional fresh parsley.

Enjoy!

PURPLE PESTO PASTA

INGREDIENTS

1 pound of pasta
of your choice

1/2 cup of fresh
basil leaves

1/4 cup of fresh purple
basil leaves

1/4 cup of freshly
grated parmesan
cheese

1/4 cup of pine nuts

2 cloves of garlic

1/4 cup of purple
sweet potatoes,
peeled and diced

1/4 cup of purple carrot,
peeled and diced

1/4 cup of purple
grapes, halved

1/4 cup of purple beet,
peeled and diced

1/4 cup of extra virgin
olive oil

Salt and pepper,
to taste

DIRECTIONS

1. Cook the pasta according to the package instructions until al dente. Drain and set aside.

2. In a blender or food processor, combine the basil leaves, purple basil leaves, parmesan cheese, pine nuts, garlic, purple sweet potatoes, purple carrot, purple grapes, purple beet, and olive oil. Blend until smooth.

3. Season with salt and pepper to taste.

4. In a large pan, toss the pasta with the pesto sauce and cook over medium heat for 2-3 minutes.

5. Serve in bowls and garnish with additional parmesan cheese and purple basil leaves.

PURPLE STUFFED PORTOBELLO MUSHROOMS

INGREDIENTS

4 large Portobello mushrooms, stems removed

1 cup cooked quinoa

1/2 cup diced purple onion

1/2 cup diced purple bell pepper

1/2 cup diced purple eggplant

2 cloves of garlic, minced

1/4 cup chopped fresh parsley

1/4 cup chopped fresh thyme

1/4 cup chopped fresh purple basil

1/4 cup grated parmesan cheese

1/4 cup breadcrumbs

2 tablespoons olive oil

Salt and pepper, to taste

DIRECTIONS

1. Preheat the oven to 375°F (190°C). Line a baking sheet with parchment paper.

2. In a skillet over medium heat, add 1 tablespoon of olive oil. Once hot, add diced purple onion, diced purple bell pepper, diced purple eggplant and garlic, cook for about 5-7 minutes or until vegetables are tender.

3. Remove from heat and mix in cooked quinoa, chopped parsley, thyme, purple basil, parmesan cheese and breadcrumbs. Season with salt and pepper to taste.

4. Brush the mushroom caps with the remaining olive oil and season with salt and pepper.

5. Stuff the mushroom caps with the quinoa mixture, dividing it evenly among the caps.

6. Place the mushrooms on the prepared baking sheet and bake for 20-25 minutes or until mushrooms are tender.

7. Serve warm.

BLACK

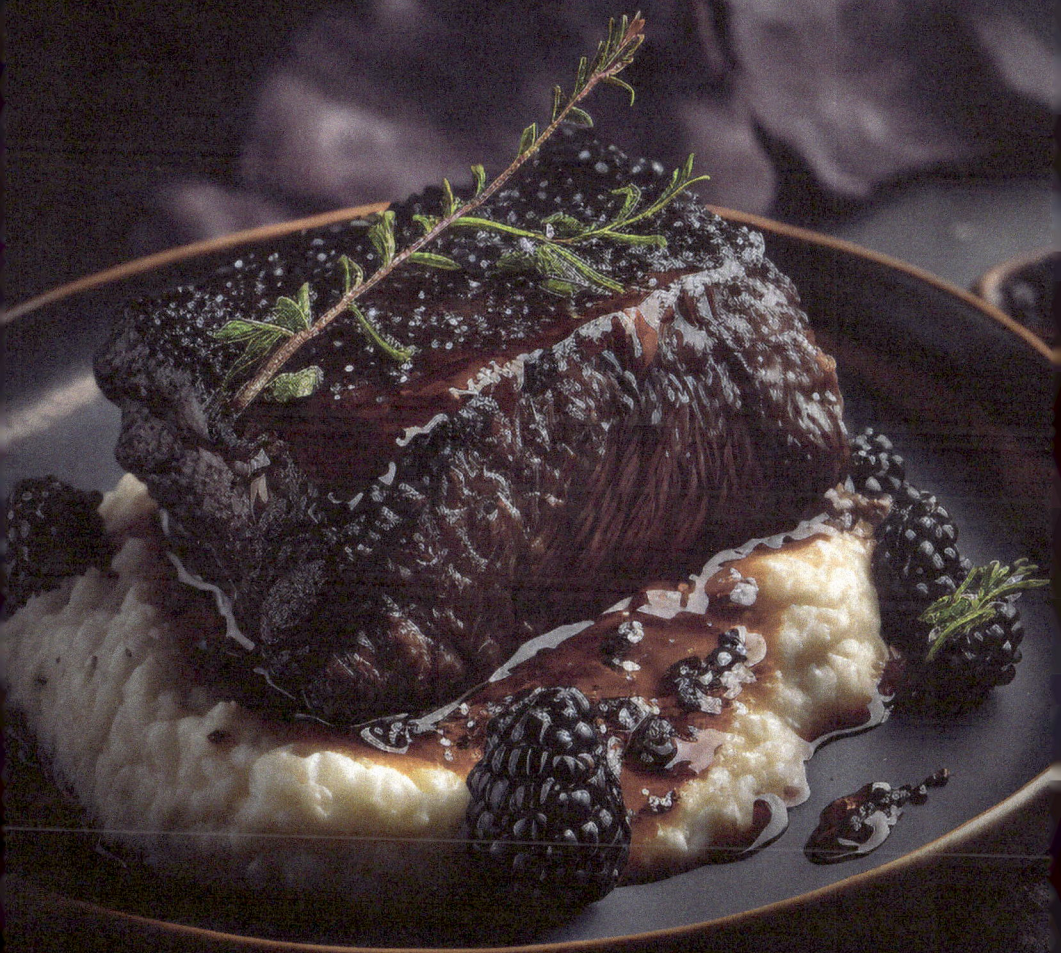

BLACKBERRY-BRAISED SHORT RIBS
WITH BLACK GARLIC MASHED POTATOES

BLACKBERRY-BRAISED SHORT RIBS WITH BLACK GARLIC MASHED POTATOES

INGREDIENTS

4 beef short ribs

2 cups beef broth

1 cup red wine

1 cup fresh blackberries

1 onion, diced

2 cloves of garlic, minced

2 sprigs of thyme

1 bay leaf

1 teaspoon salt

1/2 teaspoon black pepper

2 tablespoons olive oil

1 pound potatoes, peeled and diced

3 cloves of black garlic, minced

1/4 cup heavy cream

2 tablespoons chopped fresh parsley

DIRECTIONS

1. Preheat oven to 325 degrees F.

2. In a large Dutch oven or oven-proof pot, heat olive oil over medium-high heat. Season the short ribs with 1/2 teaspoon of salt and 1/4 teaspoon of pepper. Brown the short ribs on all sides for about 5 minutes per side.

3. Remove the short ribs from the pot and set them aside.

4. Add the onions to the pot and cook until softened, about 5 minutes. Add the garlic, thyme, bay leaf, and blackberries and cook for another 2 minutes.

5. Pour the beef broth and red wine into the pot and bring to a simmer.

6. Return the short ribs to the pot, making sure they are submerged in the liquid. Cover the pot with a lid and transfer it to the oven.

7. Braise the short ribs for 3 hours, or until they are tender and falling off the bone.

8. While the short ribs are cooking, make the black garlic mashed potatoes. In a large pot, bring the potatoes to a boil in salted water. Cook until they are tender, about 15 minutes. Drain the potatoes and return them to the pot.

9. Mash the potatoes with black garlic, heavy cream, and 1/2 teaspoon of salt. Keep warm until ready to serve.

10. Remove the short ribs from the pot and place them on a serving platter. Discard the thyme sprigs and bay leaf.

11. Strain the sauce through a fine mesh sieve and return the sauce to the pot. Bring the sauce to a boil and reduce it by half.

12. Serve the short ribs with the black garlic mashed potatoes and the reduced sauce spooned over the top. Garnish with chopped fresh parsley.

This recipe is a hearty and flavorful meal that is perfect for a special occasion or a cozy dinner at home. The blackberries add a nice sweetness to the rich and savory short ribs, while the black garlic mashed potatoes provide a unique and earthy flavor. Black Garlic is a fermented garlic that has a sweet, syrupy and complex flavor, it pairs well with the short ribs. The short ribs are a great source of protein, iron, and zinc and the potatoes a good source of potassium and Vitamin C.

BLACKBERRY-STUFFED BELL PEPPERS WITH ROSEMARY-ROASTED POTATOES

INGREDIENTS

4 large bell peppers (any color)

2 cups cooked quinoa

2 cups fresh blackberries

1/2 cup crumbled feta cheese

1/4 cup chopped fresh parsley

2 cloves of garlic, minced

1 teaspoon salt

1/2 teaspoon black pepper

1/4 cup olive oil

1/4 cup balsamic vinegar

2 tablespoons honey

1 teaspoon Dijon mustard

1 teaspoon chopped fresh rosemary

1 pound baby potatoes

DIRECTIONS

1. Preheat the oven to 375 degrees F. Line a baking sheet with parchment paper.

2. Cut the tops off the bell peppers and remove the seeds. Place the peppers on the prepared baking sheet and roast for 15 minutes, or until they start to soften.

3. In a large bowl, combine quinoa, blackberries, feta cheese, parsley, garlic, 1/2 teaspoon of salt, and 1/4 teaspoon of pepper. Mix well.

4. Remove the peppers from the oven and stuff them with the quinoa mixture. Return the peppers to the oven and bake for an additional 15 minutes, or until the peppers are fully cooked and the filling is hot.

5. While the peppers are cooking, prepare the rosemary-roasted potatoes. In a small bowl, whisk together olive oil, balsamic vinegar, honey, Dijon mustard, rosemary, 1/2 teaspoon of salt, and 1/4 teaspoon of pepper.

6. Cut the potatoes in half and toss them in the marinade. Spread the potatoes on the baking sheet and roast for 20 minutes, or until golden brown and tender.

7. Serve the stuffed peppers with rosemary-roasted potatoes on the side.

This recipe is a hearty and flavorful meal that is packed with nutrients. The combination of quinoa and blackberries makes for a delicious and healthy filling for the bell peppers. The rosemary-roasted potatoes add a nice herbaceous flavor and a crispy texture. The feta cheese add a tangy and creamy contrast to the dish. The bell peppers and blackberries are an excellent source of Vitamin C, and the quinoa provides a good source of protein and minerals like magnesium, manganese, and phosphorus.

BLACKBERRY-GLAZED EGGPLANT WITH SAGE-INFUSED QUINOA

INGREDIENTS

2 medium eggplants

2 cups fresh blackberries

2 tablespoons honey

1 tablespoon balsamic vinegar

1 teaspoon salt

1/2 teaspoon black pepper

1/4 cup olive oil

1/4 cup chopped fresh sage

1/4 teaspoon red pepper flakes

1 cup quinoa

2 cups chicken or vegetable broth

2 cloves of garlic, minced

2 scallions, thinly sliced

1/4 cup crumbled feta cheese (optional)

DIRECTIONS

1. Preheat oven to 425 degrees F. Line a baking sheet with parchment paper.

2. Cut eggplants into 1/2-inch-thick slices. Place on prepared baking sheet, and brush with 2 tablespoons of olive oil. Sprinkle with 1/2 teaspoon of salt and 1/4 teaspoon of pepper. Roast for 15 minutes, flipping halfway through, until tender and golden brown.

3. In a small saucepan, combine blackberries, honey, balsamic vinegar, and 1/4 teaspoon of salt. Cook over medium heat, stirring occasionally, until the blackberries have broken down and the mixture is thickened, about 10 minutes.

4. In a separate pan, heat remaining olive oil over medium heat. Add garlic, sage, and red pepper flakes. Cook for 1-2 minutes, until fragrant.

5. Add quinoa and chicken broth and bring to a boil. Reduce heat to low, cover, and simmer for 18 minutes, or until all the liquid is absorbed.

6. Remove quinoa from heat and let it sit, covered, for 5 minutes. Fluff with a fork and stir in scallions.

7. To assemble, place a serving of quinoa on each plate, top with eggplant slices, and spoon blackberry glaze over eggplant. Sprinkle with crumbled feta cheese, if desired. Serve immediately.

This meal is a perfect combination of sweet, savory, and spicy flavors, with the blackberry glaze adding a touch of sweetness to the eggplant, while the sage-infused quinoa provides a nice earthy contrast. The feta cheese adds a nice saltiness to the dish. The eggplant provides a good source of dietary fiber, Vitamin B1, and Vitamin B6 and quinoa a good source of protein and minerals like magnesium, manganese, and phosphorus.

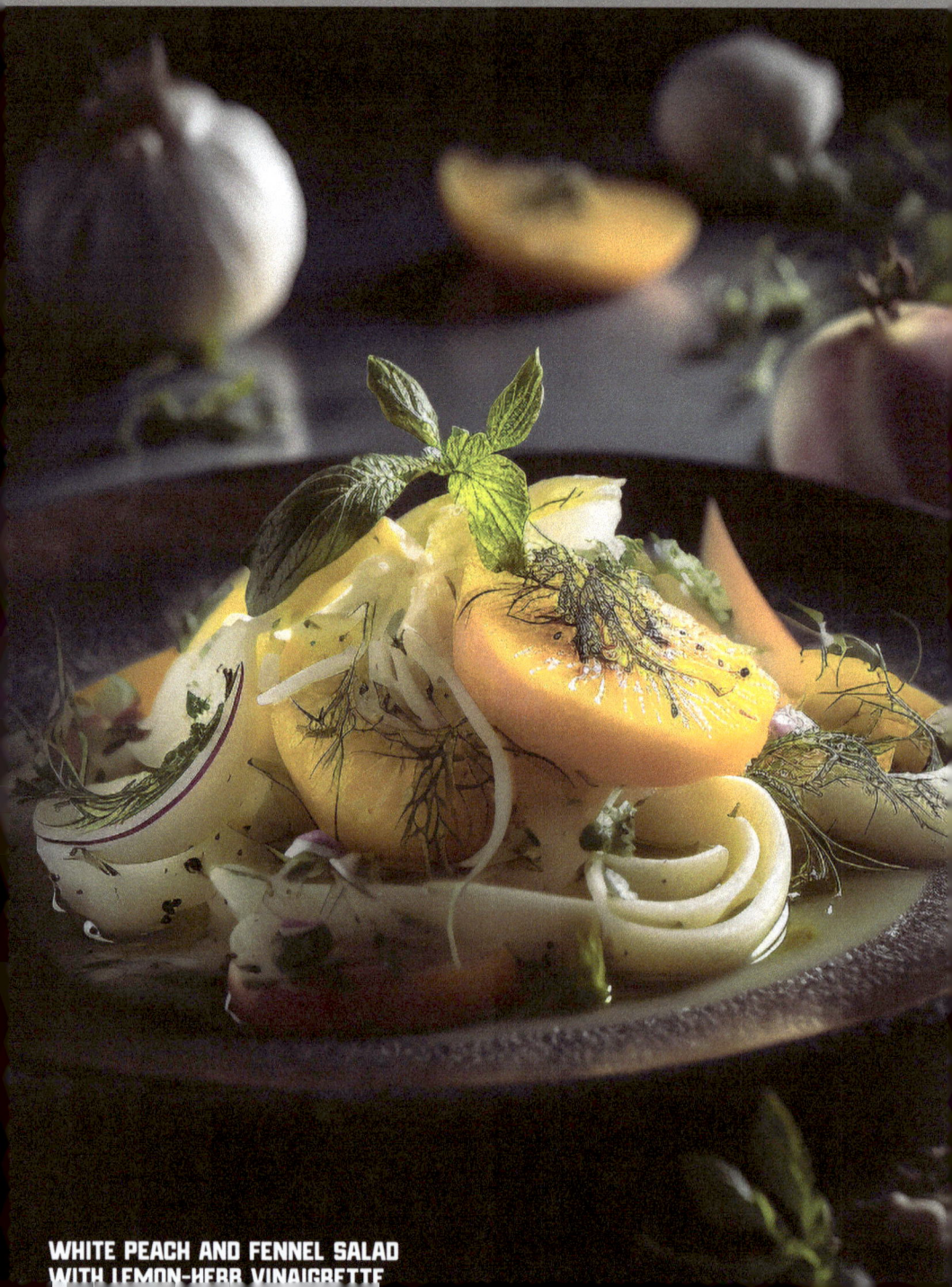

WHITE

WHITE PEACH AND FENNEL SALAD
WITH LEMON-HERB VINAIGRETTE

WHITE PEACH AND FENNEL SALAD WITH LEMON-HERB VINAIGRETTE

INGREDIENTS

2 medium fennel bulbs, thinly sliced

2 white peaches, thinly sliced

1/4 cup fresh mint leaves, chopped

1/4 cup fresh basil leaves, chopped

2 tablespoons fresh lemon juice

1 tablespoon honey

2 teaspoons Dijon mustard

1/4 cup extra-virgin olive oil

Salt and pepper, to taste

DIRECTIONS

1. In a large bowl, combine the fennel and peaches.

2. In a small bowl, whisk together the mint, basil, lemon juice, honey, Dijon mustard, and olive oil. Season with salt and pepper.

3. Drizzle the vinaigrette over the fennel and peaches, and toss to coat.

4. Serve immediately or chill in the refrigerator for at least 30 minutes before serving.

Optional: you can add some nuts or cheese like pinenuts or parmesan. Enjoy your delicious and healthy meal!

CREAMY GARLIC MUSHROOM AND POTATO SOUP

INGREDIENTS

2 tablespoons butter

1 onion, diced

4 cloves of garlic, minced

1 pound white mushrooms, sliced

2 cups chicken broth

2 cups milk

2 cups diced potatoes

1/4 cup chopped parsley

1/4 cup chopped chives

1/4 cup sour cream

Salt and pepper, to taste

DIRECTIONS

1. In a large pot or Dutch oven, melt the butter over medium heat. Add the onion and garlic and sauté until softened, about 5 minutes.

2. Add the mushrooms and cook until they release their liquid and start to brown, about 8 minutes.

3. Stir in the chicken broth, milk and potatoes. Bring to a simmer and cook until the potatoes are tender, about 15 minutes.

4. Remove from the heat and stir in the parsley and chives.

5. Use an immersion blender to puree the soup until smooth.

6. Stir in the sour cream and season with salt and pepper to taste.

7. Serve hot and garnish with additional chopped herbs if desired.

Optional: you can add some bacon or sausage for more flavor. Enjoy your creamy and comforting soup!

LEMON AND PARMESAN RISOTTO WITH WHITE ASPARAGUS AND PEAS

INGREDIENTS

1 cup Arborio rice

4 cups chicken or vegetable broth

1/2 cup white wine

1/2 cup grated Parmesan cheese

2 tablespoons butter

1/4 cup chopped shallots

2 cloves of garlic, minced

1 bunch white asparagus, trimmed and chopped

1 cup peas (fresh or frozen)

2 tablespoons chopped parsley

2 tablespoons chopped chives

1 tablespoon lemon zest

Salt and pepper, to taste

DIRECTIONS

1. In a medium saucepan, bring the broth to a simmer.

2. In a large saucepan or Dutch oven, melt the butter over medium heat. Add the shallots and garlic and sauté until softened, about 5 minutes.

3. Add the rice and stir until it becomes translucent, about 2 minutes.

4. Pour in the white wine and stir until it has been absorbed by the rice.

5. Slowly ladle in the simmering broth, one cup at a time, stirring constantly until each cup of broth has been absorbed before adding the next. This process should take about 20-25 minutes.

6. Stir in the asparagus, peas, parsley, chives and lemon zest. Cook for an additional 5 minutes or until the vegetables are tender.

7. Stir in the Parmesan cheese and season with salt and pepper to taste.

8. Serve hot and garnish with additional Parmesan cheese and herbs if desired.

Enjoy your delicious and comforting risotto!

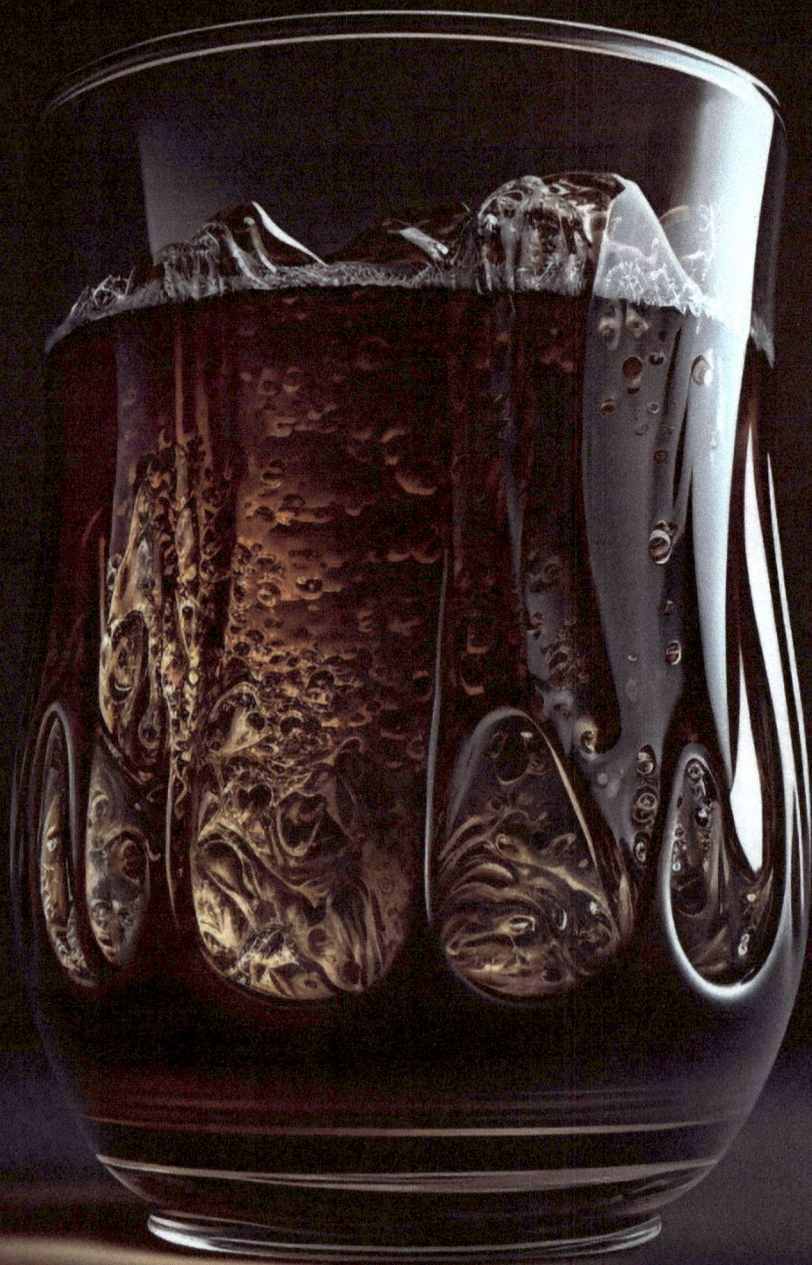

TONY'S HOMEMADE ROOT BEER

TONY'S HOMEMADE ROOT BEER

This is a real Root Beer inspired by my native roots but with some modern add-ins such as the demerara sugar.

This will make a syrup which you would mix with club soda to make your own carbonated drink.

INGREDIENTS

Sassafras Root
40 g. -or- 1.4 oz.

Sarsaparilla Root
15 g. -or- .5 oz.

Cinnamon Pieces
5 g. -or- .2 oz.

Licorice Root
10 g. -or- .35 oz.

Gentian Root
1 g. -or- .04 oz.

Demerara Sugar
450 g. -or- 16 oz.

Water (Distilled)
1000 g. -or- 35.26 oz.

DIRECTIONS

1. Add all ingredients into a pot

2. Boil till water is dissolved and solution turns syrupy

3. Turn off heat

4. Let steep 10-20 minutes

5. Let cool

6. Strain liquid

7. Pour into a air tight bottle

8. Put in refrigerator for at least 3 hours

WHEN READY TO DRINK

1 part syrup

3 parts club soda

Stir until mixed

Drink and enjoy

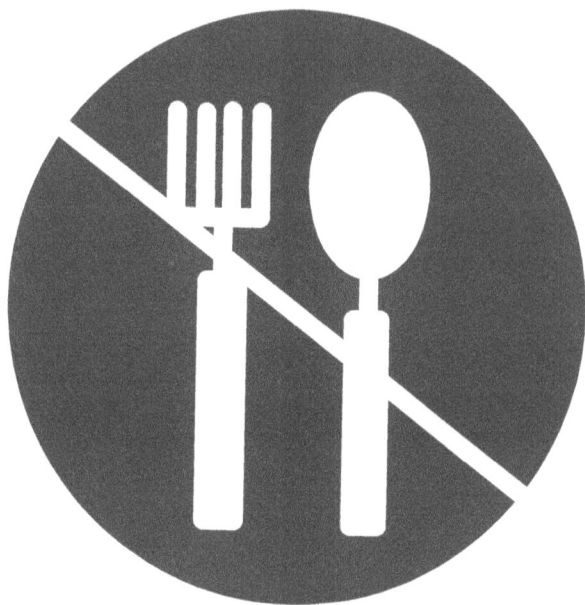

THE BENEFITS OF FASTING

Although fasting has become ever more popular for improving your health and wellness, it is an age-old practice and plays a significant part in several religions and cultures. Fasting means abstaining or limiting all or some foods or drinks for a predetermined time.

There are numerous ways to fast. In general, most fasts last between 12 and 72 hours. Intermittent fasting, on the other hand, comprises cycling between eating and fasting stages that can last anywhere from a few hours to a few days.

Fasting can give several health benefits, from weight reduction to improved cognitive function.

First, let's have a look at how to start fasting.

HOW TO START FASTING

There are many forms of fasts, making it simple to pick one that works for you.

The following are some of the most prevalent types of fasting:

- Water fasting entails only drinking water for a specific time.

- Juice fasting entails drinking just vegetable or fruit juice for a set amount of time.

- Intermittent fasting, in which intake is restricted for a few hours to a few days at a time, with a standard diet resumed on other days. It is employed in several cultural, religious, and personal contexts.

- Partial fasting is when certain foods or drinks, such as processed foods, animal products, or caffeine, are removed from the diet for a set period.

- Calorie restriction means that calories are restricted for a few days every week.

- and, The New Rainbow Fast created by Tony Vortex to help with specific ailments, or goals.

There are even more types of fasts within these categories, such as intermittent fasting, which can be divided into subcategories such as alternate-day fasting, which includes intake every other day, or time-restricted feeding, which requires eating only a few hours per day and restricting intake the rest of the time.

FASTING IN MUSLIM COUNTRIES: A widespread religious practice is intermittent fasts which involve avoiding any food or drinks from early morning to early evening and having all sorts of foods during the rest of the day, which is presumed to impart numerous health benefits with spiritual aspects.

The exact mechanism of how it enhances health is unknown; however, some theories from scientific studies are of the view that it involves the reduction in the production of reactive oxidative species, increased ketosis, and optimization of central and peripheral circadian physiological processes.

FASTING AND INDIAN CULTURE: Fasting as a spiritual and moral act is an essential element of Hinduism for purifying the mind and body and acquiring divine grace. It can range from mild restriction to complete abstinence, such as you may abstain from just one meal in a day, or avoid a particular food type, or you can be more strict. Fasting days and methods are not imposed but are determined by the community, family, or individual.

To begin, experiment with different types of fasting to see what works best for you according to your health, dietary habits, and lifestyle. Consulting a nutritionist or physician can be a better option in this regard.

HEALTH BENEFITS OF FASTING

Fasting has been linked to various health benefits, including:

- Enhanced weight management

- Better blood sugar control

- Reduced inflammation

- Improved heart health

- May also protect against diseases like cancer and neurological illnesses

ENHANCES HEALTH
BY COMBATING INFLAMMATION

While acute inflammation is a natural immune response used to help fight infections, chronic inflammation can have significant health repercussions. According to research, chronic inflammation may play a role in developing severe illnesses such as heart disease, cancer, and rheumatoid arthritis.

Fasting has been proven in numerous studies to aid in reducing inflammation and promoting improved health. A meta-analysis of 18 research discovered that intermittent fasting could considerably lower C-reactive protein levels, a measure of inflammation.

Another small study revealed that adopting intermittent fasting for a year was more successful than a control group at lowering inflammation and some risk factors for heart disease.

Furthermore, one animal study discovered that eating a very low-calorie diet to simulate the effects of fasting reduced inflammation and was influential in treating multiple sclerosis, a chronic inflammatory disorder.

IMPROVES HEART HEALTH
BY LOWERING BLOOD PRESSURE,
LIPIDS, AND CHOLESTEROL

Heart disease is the leading cause of death worldwide, accounting for an estimated 31.5% of all deaths. One of the most effective ways to minimize cardiovascular disease risk is to modify your dietary pattern and lifestyle.

Based on certain studies, it has been concluded that including fasting in your regimen can be very beneficial for your heart health. One study found that, compared to a control group, alternate-day fasting could lower total cholesterol levels and numerous risk factors for heart disease in adults who are overweight.

Another study found that alternate-day fasting significantly reduced blood pressure and blood triglycerides, total cholesterol, and LDL (bad) cholesterol levels.

Furthermore, an older study of 4,629 adults linked fasting to a lower risk of coronary artery disease as well as a significantly lower chance of diabetes, which is a significant risk factor for heart disease.

IT LESSENS INSULIN RESISTANCE AND IMPROVES CONTROL OF BLOOD SUGAR

Several studies have suggested that fasting improves blood sugar control, which could be especially beneficial for people with diabetes. Research involving ten type-2 diabetic patients demonstrated that short-term intermittent fasting lowered blood sugar levels significantly.

Meanwhile, another 2014 study discovered that intermittent and alternate-day fasting were equally efficient at reducing insulin resistance as calorie restriction.

Reduced insulin resistance can enhance your body's sensitivity to insulin, moving glucose more efficiently from your bloodstream to your cells.

Combined with the potential blood sugar-lowering impacts of fasting, this could help keep your blood sugar stable, reducing blood sugar spikes and crashes.

However, other studies have indicated that fasting affects blood sugar levels and insulin resistance differently in men and women. For example, one older 3-week trial found that alternate-day fasting harmed female blood sugar regulation but did not affect males.

IT HELPS WITH WEIGHT LOSS BY DECREASING CALORIE INTAKE AND INCREASING METABOLISM

Many dieters try fasting to reduce weight. In theory, avoiding all or certain foods and beverages should reduce your overall calorie consumption, potentially leading to increased weight loss over time.

In animal studies, short-term fasting promotes metabolism by boosting levels of the neurotransmitter norepinephrine, which may aid in weight loss. One study found that fasting for the entire day could reduce body weight by up to 9% and considerably reduce body fat over 12-24 weeks.

Another study discovered intermittent fasting was more efficient than constant calorie restriction in causing weight loss. Furthermore, several studies have demonstrated that fasting may significantly reduce body and belly fat more than ongoing calorie restriction.

IT MAY IMPROVE BRAIN FUNCTION AND HELP TO PREVENT NEURO-DEGENERATIVE DISEASES

Though most studies have been conducted on animals, some investigations have discovered that fasting may significantly impact brain function.

In a 2013 study on mice, intermittent fasting for 11 months increased brain function and anatomy. Other animal research has found that fasting can improve cognitive function by protecting brain health and increasing nerve cell production.

Fasting, as already discussed, may also help alleviate inflammation, which may aid in the prevention of neurodegenerative illnesses.

Fasting, in particular, appears to protect against and improve results in animal tests for illnesses such as Alzheimer's and Parkinson's.

Some religious beliefs in several Muslim countries are of the view that fasting improves memory. It has also been highlighted in a systematic review study published in the Journal of Pakistan Medical Association in 2019 that demonstrated that Islamic fasting, which involves the complete prohibition of any food or drinks from dawn to dusk, has a positive impact on cognitive activities such as visual memory, spatial memory, and attention.

INCREASES THE SECRETION OF GROWTH HORMONE, WHICH IS ESSENTIAL FOR DEVELOPMENT, METABOLISM, WEIGHT LOSS, AND MUSCLE STRENGTH

The protein hormone human growth factor (HGH) plays a crucial role in various areas of your health. Indeed, research indicates that this vital hormone is involved in metabolism, weight reduction, and muscular growth.

Fasting has been revealed in more than a few research studies to boost the levels of HGH naturally. Fasting for 24 hours dramatically raised HGH levels in one study of 11 healthy adults. Another small, older study of nine males discovered that fasting for just two days increased HGH synthesis by fivefold.

Furthermore, as mentioned earlier, fasting may help maintain consistent blood sugar and insulin levels throughout the day, which may assist in optimizing HGH levels further, as some study has revealed that insulin can influence HGH output.

HOW CANCER PREVENTION AND CHEMOTHERAPY EFFECTIVENESS MAY BE IMPROVED

Fasting appears to aid cancer treatment and prevention in animal and test-tube research. An older study discovered that fasting on alternate days helped to prevent tumor growth. Several animal and test-tube studies also believe fasting could lessen tumor progression and increase chemotherapy effectiveness.

Unfortunately, most of these studies on the impact of fasting on cancer formation are limited to cell studies. Hence, despite these encouraging findings, more research is needed to determine how fasting may influence cancer growth and therapy in humans.

COULD DELAY AGING AND ENHANCE LONGEVITY

Animal research on the possible lifespan-extension effects of fasting has yielded promising results. In one study, rats who fasted lived 28% longer and acquired disease 28% later than rats with unlimited food access.

Other studies have found similar results, indicating that fasting may help improve longevity and delay the disease.

However, most current research is confined to animal studies. More studies about how fasting affects aging and longevity in humans may be needed.

THE RAINBOW FAST

The food that we eat is so nourishing for our bodies that in my opinion, all that we have to do is take the time to listen. Listening in this case also means not abusing the body by subjecting it to toxic substances, constantly doing over-stressing activities, and not allowing it the needed time to rejuvenate.

Each color of the rainbow (in relation to the food) has its specific benefits which include:

BLACK

To boost the immune system and increase antioxidant levels to fight off the illness

WHITE

To reduce inflammation and provide essential vitamins and minerals to support recovery

VIOLET/PURPLE

To protect against chronic disease and boost the immune system

BLUE/INDIGO

To promote heart health, improve brain function, aid digestion, and support the skin while recovering.

GREEN

To reduce the risk of chronic diseases, promoting a healthy gut and immune system, and to aid weight management and hydration to support recovery

YELLOW

To promote digestion, support the immune system, and improve skin health.

ORANGE

To support healthy vision, boost the immune system, and promote healthy skin and digestion.

RED

To support heart health, reduce the risk of certain cancers, boost the immune system, and promote healthy skin.

When I created this fast back in the year 2005 I experimented with the most healthiest way to receive the benefits of the color in question with the optimal life style change as not to hurt myself.

Based on the trials I undertook and the family and friends who also went along on this journey with me as I was figuring out the best approach, this is what I suggest:

- Do not consume a color more than one week in length.
  But you are welcome to alternate between colors week after week.

- For example, the first week you may do green,
  but then the next blue, the next orange etc.

- These mono weekly color changes should not extend
  past 60 days (8 weeks) in length total.

I have done a total of 6 months (approximately 180 days) on various versions of the rainbow fast with zero issues. But at that time I was young, very healthy, athletic and active. One time I went 60 days just on Blue / Indigo fruits, vegetables and herbs only, which to this day was the only time that I was sleeping a maximum of 4 hours a night and completely rested, with zero fatigue or needing to take a rest midday. This effect lasted for over a year.

Our bodies have a basic design which makes the underlying premise to health easy and routine, but then there are those overreaching differences which one has to consider. What worked for me, may not work for you and vice-versa.

Take your time, you now have this manual in your hands and you can come back to it as needed.

Also I host events yearly about many different subjects which many are welcome to attend and my contact information is at the back of this book if a question arises.

PRECAUTIONS ASSOCIATED WITH FASTING

Although fasting offers many health benefits, it is still not recommended or appropriate for everyone. Fasting, for example, can cause severe rises and dips in blood sugar levels if you have diabetes.

If you have any underlying health concerns or want to fast for more than 24 hours, you should consult a doctor first.

Fasting is also not generally advised without medical supervision for elderly adults, adolescents, or underweight persons.

To maximize the potential health benefits of fasting, remain hydrated and enrich your diet with nutrient-dense foods throughout your feeding intervals.

Also, if fasting for an extended period, try to avoid strenuous physical activity and get plenty of rest.

THE TAKEAWAY

The practice of fasting has been linked to a wide range of potential health benefits, including weight loss, improved blood sugar control, enhanced heart health, better brain function, and cancer prevention.

Numerous fasting styles accommodate practically every lifestyle, from water fasting to intermittent fasting and calorie restriction.

Fasting may help your health when combined with a balanced diet and a healthy lifestyle to live a long, disease free life.

REFERENCES:

- Ojha U, Khanal S, Park PH, Hong JT, Choi DY. Intermittent fasting protects the nigral dopaminergic neurons from MPTP-mediated dopaminergic neuronal injury in mice. J Nutr Biochem. 2022 Nov 10;112:109212. doi: 10.1016/j.jnutbio.2022.109212. Epub ahead of print. PMID: 36370926.

- Nasaruddin ML, Syed Abd Halim SA, Kamaruzzaman MA. Studying the Relationship of Intermittent Fasting and β-Amyloid in Animal Model of Alzheimer's Disease: A Scoping Review. Nutrients. 2020 Oct 21;12(10):3215. doi: 10.3390/nu12103215. PMID: 33096730; PMCID: PMC7590153.

- Shin BK, Kang S, Kim DS, Park S. Intermittent fasting protects against the deterioration of cognitive function, energy metabolism and dyslipidemia in Alzheimer's disease-induced estrogen deficient rats. Exp Biol Med (Maywood). 2018 Feb;243(4):334-343. doi: 10.1177/1535370217751610. Epub 2018 Jan 7. PMID: 29307281; PMCID: PMC6022926.

- Elesawy BH, Raafat BM, Muqbali AA, Abbas AM, Sakr HF. The Impact of Intermittent Fasting on Brain-Derived Neurotrophic Factor, Neurotrophin 3, and Rat Behavior in a Rat Model of Type 2 Diabetes Mellitus. Brain Sci. 2021 Feb 15;11(2):242. doi: 10.3390/brainsci11020242. PMID: 33671898; PMCID: PMC7918995.

- Li L, Wang Z, Zuo Z. Chronic intermittent fasting improves cognitive functions and brain structures in mice. PLoS One. 2013 Jun 3;8(6):e66069. doi: 10.1371/journal.pone.0066069. PMID: 23755298; PMCID: PMC3670843.

- Tinsley GM, La Bounty PM. Effects of intermittent fasting on body composition and clinical health markers in humans. Nutr Rev. 2015 Oct;73(10):661-74. doi: 10.1093/nutrit/nuv041. Epub 2015 Sep 15. PMID: 26374764.

- Zhang Q, Zhang C, Wang H, Ma Z, Liu D, Guan X, Liu Y, Fu Y, Cui M, Dong J. Intermittent Fasting versus Continuous Calorie Restriction: Which Is Better for Weight Loss? Nutrients. 2022 Apr 24;14(9):1781. doi: 10.3390/nu14091781. PMID: 35565749; PMCID: PMC9099935.

- Enríquez Guerrero A, San Mauro Martín I, Garicano Vilar E, Camina Martín MA. Effectiveness of an intermittent fasting diet versus continuous energy restriction on anthropometric measurements, body composition and lipid profile in overweight and obese adults: a meta-analysis. Eur J Clin Nutr. 2021 Jul;75(7):1024-1039. doi: 10.1038/s41430-020-00821-1. Epub 2020 Dec 9. PMID: 33293678.

- Hjelholt A, Høgild M, Bak AM, Arlien-Søborg MC, Bæk A, Jessen N, Richelsen B, Pedersen SB, Møller N, Lunde Jørgensen JO. Growth Hormone and Obesity. Endocrinol Metab Clin North Am. 2020 Jun;49(2):239-250. doi: 10.1016/j.ecl.2020.02.009. Epub 2020 Apr 16. PMID: 32418587.

- Fink J, Schoenfeld BJ, Nakazato K. The role of hormones in muscle hypertrophy. Phys Sportsmed. 2018 Feb;46(1):129-134. doi: 10.1080/00913847.2018.1406778. Epub 2017 Nov 25. PMID: 29172848.

- Salgin B, Marcovecchio ML, Hill N, Dunger DB, Frystyk J. The effect of prolonged fasting on levels of growth hormone-binding protein and free growth hormone. Growth Horm IGF Res. 2012 Apr;22(2):76-81. doi: 10.1016/j.ghir.2012.02.003. Epub 2012 Mar 3. PMID: 22386777.

- Hartman ML, Veldhuis JD, Johnson ML, Lee MM, Alberti KG, Samojlik E, Thorner MO. Augmented growth hormone (GH) secretory burst frequency and amplitude mediate enhanced GH secretion during a two-day fast in normal men. J Clin Endocrinol Metab. 1992 Apr;74(4):757-65. doi: 10.1210/jcem.74.4.1548337. PMID: 1548337.

- Qiu H, Yang JK, Chen C. Influence of insulin on growth hormone secretion, level and growth hormone signaling. Sheng Li Xue Bao. 2017 Oct 25;69(5):541-556. PMID: 29063103.

- Gotthardt JD, Verpeut JL, Yeomans BL, Yang JA, Yasrebi A, Roepke TA, Bello NT. Intermittent Fasting Promotes Fat Loss With Lean MassRetention, Increased Hypothalamic Norepinephrine Content, and Increased Neuropeptide Y Gene Expression in Diet-Induced Obese Male Mice. Endocrinology. 2016 Feb;157(2):679-91. doi: 10.1210/en.2015-1622. Epub 2015 Dec 14. PMID: 26653760; PMCID: PMC4733124.

- Pourabbasi A, Ebrahimnegad Shirvani MS, Shams AH. Does Islamic fasting affect cognitive functions in adolescents? A systematic review. J Pak Med Assoc. 2019 Aug;69(8):1164-1169. PMID: 31431772.

• Rocha NS, Barbisan LF, de Oliveira ML, de Camargo JL. Effects of fasting and intermittent fasting on rat hepatocarcinogenesis induced by diethylnitrosamine. Teratog Carcinog Mutagen. 2002;22(2):129-38. doi: 10.1002/tcm.10005. PMID: 11835290.

• Clifton KK, Ma CX, Fontana L, Peterson LL. Intermittent fasting in the prevention and treatment of cancer. CA Cancer J Clin. 2021 Nov;71(6):527-546. doi: 10.3322/caac.21694. Epub 2021 Aug 12. PMID: 34383300.

• Sadeghian M, Rahmani S, Khalesi S, Hejazi E. A review of fasting effects on the response of cancer to chemotherapy. Clin Nutr. 2021 Apr;40(4):1669-1681. doi: 10.1016/j.clnu.2020.10.037. Epub 2020 Oct 23. PMID: 33153820.

• Mitchell SJ, Bernier M, Mattison JA, Aon MA, Kaiser TA, Anson RM, Ikeno Y, Anderson RM, Ingram DK, de Cabo R. Daily Fasting Improves Health and Survival in Male Mice Independent of Diet Composition and Calories. Cell Metab. 2019 Jan 8;29(1):221-228.e3. doi: 10.1016/j.cmet.2018.08.011. Epub 2018 Sep 6. PMID: 30197301; PMCID: PMC6326845.

• Longo VD, Di Tano M, Mattson MP, Guidi N. Intermittent and periodic fasting, longevity, and disease. Nat Aging. 2021 Jan;1(1):47-59.doi: 10.1038/s43587-020-00013-3. Epub 2021 Jan 14. PMID: 35310455; PMCID: PMC8932957.

• Arnason TG, Bowen MW, Mansell KD. Effects of intermittent fasting on health markers in those with type 2 diabetes: A pilot study. World J Diabetes. 2017 Apr 15;8(4):154-164. doi: 10.4239/wjd.v8.i4.154. PMID: 28465792; PMCID: PMC5394735.

• Barnosky AR, Hoddy KK, Unterman TG, Varady KA. Intermittent fasting vs. daily calorie restriction for type 2 diabetes prevention: a review of human findings. Transl Res. 2014 Oct;164(4):302-11. doi: 10.1016/j.trsl.2014.05.013. Epub 2014 Jun 12. PMID: 24993615.

• Heilbronn LK, Civitarese AE, Bogacka I, Smith SR, Hulver M, Ravussin E. Glucose tolerance and skeletal muscle gene expression in response to alternate day fasting. Obes Res. 2005 Mar;13(3):574-81. doi: 10.1038/oby.2005.61. PMID: 15833943.

- Moro T, Tinsley G, Pacelli FQ, Marcolin G, Bianco A, Paoli A. Twelve Months of Time-restricted Eating and Resistance Training Improves Inflammatory Markers and Cardiometabolic Risk Factors. Med Sci Sports Exerc. 2021 Dec 1;53(12):2577-2585. doi: 10.1249/MSS.0000000000002738. PMID: 34649266.

- Choi IY, Piccio L, Childress P, Bollman B, Ghosh A, Brandhorst S, Suarez J, Michalsen A, Cross AH, Morgan TE, Wei M, Paul F, Bock M, Longo VD. A Diet Mimicking Fasting Promotes Regeneration and Reduces Autoimmunity and Multiple Sclerosis Symptoms. Cell Rep. 2016 Jun 7;15(10):2136-2146. doi: 10.1016/j.celrep.2016.05.009. Epub 2016 May 26. PMID: 27239035; PMCID: PMC4899145.

- Heilbronn LK, Civitarese AE, Bogacka I, Smith SR, Hulver M, Ravussin E. Glucose tolerance and skeletal muscle gene expression in response to alternate day fasting. Obes Res. 2005 Mar;13(3):574-81. doi: 10.1038/oby.2005.61. PMID: 15833943.

- Horne BD, May HT, Anderson JL, Kfoury AG, Bailey BM, McClure BS, Renlund DG, Lappé DL, Carlquist JF, Fisher PW, Pearson RR, Bair TL, Adams TD, Muhlestein JB; Intermountain Heart Collaborative Study. Usefulness of routine periodic fasting to lower risk of coronary artery disease in patients undergoing coronary angiography. Am J Cardiol. 2008 Oct 1;102(7):814-819. doi: 10.1016/j.amjcard.2008.05.021. Epub 2008 Jul 10. PMID: 18805103; PMCID: PMC2572991.

- Cui Y, Cai T, Zhou Z, Mu Y, Lu Y, Gao Z, Wu J, Zhang Y. Health Effects of Alternate-Day Fasting in Adults: A Systematic Review and Meta-Analysis. Front Nutr. 2020 Nov 24;7:586036. doi: 10.3389/fnut.2020.586036. PMID: 33330587; PMCID: PMC7732631.

- Park J, Seo YG, Paek YJ, Song HJ, Park KH, Noh HM. Effect of alternate-day fasting on obesity and cardiometabolic risk: A systematic review and meta-analysis. Metabolism. 2020 Oct;111:154336. doi: 10.1016/j.metabol.2020.154336. Epub 2020 Aug 7. PMID: 32777443.

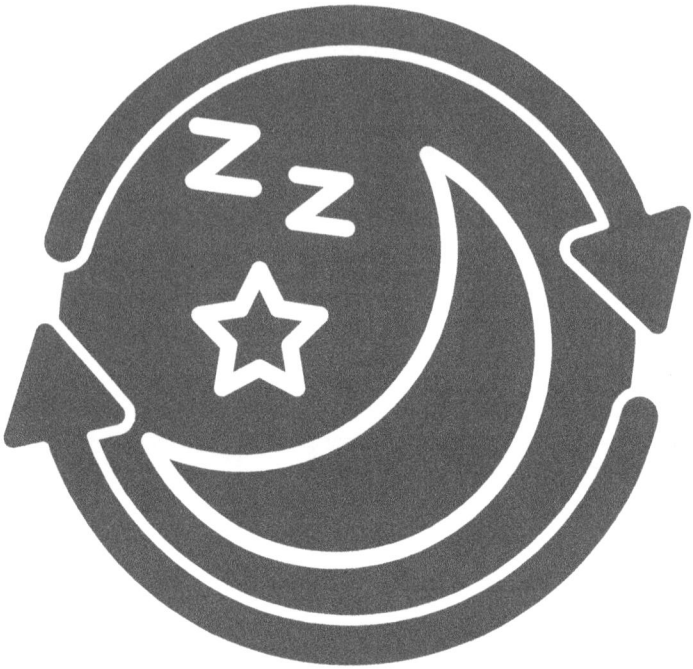

TRANSFORM YOUR SLEEP: ACHIEVING A GOOD NIGHT'S REST AND OVERCOMING SLEEP DISORDERS

The importance of a good night's sleep cannot be overstated. Sleep plays a crucial role in maintaining physical and mental health, and a lack of sleep can lead to various health problems. In this chapter, I will delve into the various aspects of sleep, including the different stages of sleep, the effects of sleep deprivation, and the underlying causes of sleep disorders.

First, it's essential to understand the different stages of sleep. Sleep is divided into two main categories: rapid-eye movement (REM) sleep and non-rapid-eye movement (NREM) sleep. NREM sleep is divided into three stages: N1, N2, and N3. Each phase serves a different purpose and is characterized by distinct brain wave patterns. During N1, the brain is in a light sleep state and is easily awakened. N2 is a deeper sleep stage where the brain's activity is slower and more synchronized. N3 is the deepest sleep stage characterized by slow brain waves, also known as delta waves. In this stage, the body repairs and regenerates tissues build bone and muscle, and strengthens the immune system.

Rapid eye movements and increased brain activity characterize REM sleep. This is the stage of sleep where most dreaming occurs. The REM stage is essential for learning, memory consolidation, and emotional regulation. A typical night's sleep cycle includes four or five cycles of NREM and REM sleep, with the longest period of deep N3 sleep occurring in the first half of the night.

Now that we have a basic understanding of the different stages of sleep let's talk about the effects of sleep deprivation. Sleep deprivation is defined as not getting enough sleep, which can have severe physical and mental health consequences. Chronic sleep deprivation has been linked to an increased risk of obesity, diabetes, cardiovascular disease, and an impaired immune system. It can also affect mood, cognitive function, and performance at work or school. Furthermore, It can increase the risk of accidents, especially drowsy driving.

One of the most severe effects of chronic sleep deprivation is cognitive impairment. Studies have shown that even a night of poor sleep can lead to decreased attention, poor memory, and poor decision-making abilities (Dinges et al., 1997). This is particularly concerning for individuals who work in safety-sensitive jobs, such as healthcare professionals, truck drivers, and pilots. Furthermore, sleep deprivation can affect emotional regulation and can lead to irritability, anxiety, and depression.

Chronic sleep deprivation can adversely affect both physical and mental health.

SOME EXAMPLES INCLUDE

- **Increased risk of obesity and diabetes:** Lack of sleep can disrupt hormones that control appetite, leading to weight gain and an increased risk of developing diabetes.

- **Cardiovascular disease:** Chronic sleep deprivation has been linked to an increased risk of heart disease, high blood pressure, and stroke.

- **Impaired immune system:** Sleep plays a vital role in maintaining the body's immune function. Chronic sleep deprivation can make individuals more susceptible to illnesses and infections.

- **Mood disorders:** Lack of sleep can lead to irritability, anxiety, and depression.

- **Cognitive impairment:** Chronic sleep deprivation can affect cognitive function, including memory, attention, and decision-making.

- **Performance deficits:** Sleep deprivation can affect performance at work or school, including reaction time, attention, and decision-making.

- **Increased risk of accidents:** Drowsy driving is a leading cause of traffic accidents and can be as dangerous as driving under the influence of alcohol.

- **Poor physical and mental well-being:** Chronic sleep deprivation can lead to fatigue, decreased motivation, and feeling unwell.

Now that we've discussed the effects of sleep deprivation let's talk about the underlying causes of sleep disorders. Sleep disorders can have multiple causes and can be complex. Medical conditions like asthma, acid reflux, and thyroid disorders can cause them. Medications, such as antidepressants and blood pressure medications, can also cause them. Environmental factors, such as noise, light, temperature, and an uncomfortable bed, can also lead to sleep problems.

Mental health conditions such as anxiety and depression are also common causes of sleep disorders. These disorders can lead to insomnia or other sleep problems. Chronic pain can also make it difficult to fall asleep or stay asleep. Additionally, sleep disorders can be caused by disruptions in the body's internal clock, known as circadian rhythm disorders. Examples of circadian rhythm disorders include jet lag, shift work sleep disorder, and delayed sleep phase syndrome.

Severe lack of sleep, also known as chronic sleep deprivation, can lead to several illnesses.

SOME EXAMPLES INCLUDE

- **Cardiovascular disease:** Chronic sleep deprivation has been linked to an increased risk of heart disease, high blood pressure, and stroke.

- **Diabetes:** Lack of sleep can disrupt hormones that control blood sugar levels, increasing the risk of developing diabetes.

- **Obesity:** Sleep plays a role in regulating hormones that control appetite, leading to weight gain if you don't get enough sleep.

- **Depression:** Chronic sleep deprivation has been linked to an increased risk of developing depression.

- **Anxiety:** Sleep plays an essential role in regulating emotions, and chronic sleep deprivation can lead to feelings of anxiety.

- **Attention Deficit Hyperactivity Disorder (ADHD):** Lack of sleep can affect attention and concentration, which can lead to symptoms of ADHD.

- **Alzheimer's disease:** Sleep plays an important role in the consolidation of memories, and chronic sleep deprivation has been linked to an increased risk of developing Alzheimer's disease.

- **Gastrointestinal issues:** Chronic sleep deprivation has been linked to gastrointestinal problems such as GERD and ulcers.

- **Weakened immune system:** Sleep plays an important role in maintaining the body's immune function. Chronic sleep deprivation can make individuals more susceptible to illnesses and infections.

Sleep is crucial for overall health and well-being. A lack of sleep can lead to various health problems, including obesity, diabetes, cardiovascular disease, and an impaired immune system. It can also affect mood, cognitive function, and performance at work or school. Sleep disorders can have multiple causes and can be complex, including medical conditions, medications, environmental factors, mental health conditions, chronic pain, and disruptions in the body's internal clock.

To ensure a good night's sleep, it's crucial to establish a regular sleep schedule, create a comfortable sleep environment, and avoid stimulating activities and substances before bedtime. Additionally, it's important to address underlying sleep disorders or health issues contributing to sleep problems.

If you have difficulty sleeping, it's important to consult a healthcare professional to determine the cause and the best course of treatment. Treatment options may include cognitive-behavioral therapy, medication, or lifestyle changes such as regular exercise, relaxation techniques, and a healthy diet.

THERE ARE SEVERAL FOODS AND TEAS THAT CAN HELP PROMOTE A GOOD NIGHT'S SLEEP WHICH INCLUDE

- **Cherries:** Cherries contain melatonin, a hormone that regulates the sleep-wake cycle. Eating cherries or drinking cherry juice before bed can help to promote sleep.

- **Bananas:** Bananas contain potassium and magnesium, which can help relax muscles and promote calmness.

- **Whole grains:** Whole grains such as oatmeal and whole wheat bread are rich in magnesium, which can help to relax muscles and promote calmness.

- **Nuts and seeds:** Nuts and seeds such as almonds, walnuts, and pumpkin seeds are rich in magnesium and tryptophan, which can help to promote sleep.

- **Herbal teas:** Herbal teas such as chamomile, valerian, and lemon balm have been used for centuries to promote sleep. These teas contain compounds that can help calm the mind and promote relaxation.

- **Honey:** Honey can help to raise insulin levels, which allows tryptophan to enter the brain more easily.

- **Fish:** Fish, particularly tuna and salmon, contain high levels of vitamin B6, which plays a crucial role in melatonin production.

A GOOD NIGHT'S SLEEP PROVIDES SEVERAL BENEFITS FOR PHYSICAL AND MENTAL HEALTH, WHICH INCLUDE

- **Improved physical health:** Sleep helps to repair and restore the body, which can help to reduce the risk of developing certain diseases such as obesity, diabetes, and heart disease.

- **Enhanced immune function:** Sleep plays an important role in maintaining the body's immune function, making you less susceptible to illnesses and infections.

- **Improved cognitive function:** Sleep helps to consolidate memories and learning, improving performance at work or school.

- **Better mood:** Sleep is essential for maintaining emotional well-being and can help reduce feelings of irritability, anxiety, and depression.

- **Increased safety:** Adequate sleep can improve reaction time, attention, and decision-making, which can help to reduce the risk of accidents, both on the job and in daily life.

- **Increased productivity:** Getting enough sleep can make you feel more energized and motivated throughout the day.

- **Better physical and mental well-being:** Adequate sleep can help you feel refreshed and rejuvenated, allowing you to face the day positively.

- **Better weight management:** Adequate sleep can help regulate hormones that control appetite and metabolism, leading to better weight management.

- **Improved athletic performance:** Adequate sleep is vital for physical recovery and can help improve athletic performance.

- **Improved memory and learning:** Sleep plays a crucial role in consolidating memories and learning, allowing the brain to process and store new information.

- **Improved skin health:** Sleep is vital for maintaining healthy skin, as the body produces collagen during sleep, which can help reduce wrinkles and improve skin elasticity.

- **Reduced stress:** Sleep can help reduce the levels of stress hormones in the body, promoting a sense of calm and relaxation.

- **Lower risk of depression:** Adequate sleep is essential for maintaining emotional well-being and can help reduce the risk of developing depression.

- **Lower risk of accidents:** Adequate sleep can improve reaction time, attention, and decision-making, which can help to reduce the risk of accidents, both on the job and in daily life.

- **Improved relationships:** Sleep plays an important role in maintaining emotional well-being, which can lead to better relationships with others.

- **Increased longevity:** A good night's sleep can improve overall health and well-being, leading to a healthier life.

As we continue to put forth the most important content for a healthy life, hopefully, those who read this innerstand that sleep is a vital component of overall health and well-being, and it's important to prioritize it and address any underlying issues that may be affecting it.

REFERENCES:

- Dinges, D. F., Pack, F., Williams, K., Gillen, K. A., Powell, J. W., Ott, G. E., & Aptowicz, C. (1997). Cumulative sleepiness, mood disturbance, and psychomotor vigilance performance decrements during a week of sleep restricted to 4—5 hours per night. Sleep, 20(4), 267— https://doi.org/10.1093/sleep/20.4.267

- National Sleep Foundation. (n.d.). Sleep and Sleep disorders. Retrieved from https://www.sleepfoundation.org/

- American Academy of Sleep Medicine. (n.d.). Sleep disorders. Retrieved from https://www.aasm.org/

- Sleep Research Society. (n.d.). Sleep research and the science of sleep. Retrieved from https://www.sleepresearchsociety.org/

- Centers for Disease Control and Prevention (CDC). (n.d.). Sleep and sleep disorders. Retrieved from https://www.cdc.gov/sleep/index.html

- National Institute of Neurological Disorders and Stroke (NINDS). (n.d.). Sleep disorders information page. Retrieved from https://www.ninds.nih.gov/Disorders/All-Disorders/Sleep-Disorders-Information-Page

- American Insomnia Association. (n.d.). Sleep disorders and insomnia. Retrieved from https://www.americaninsomniaassociation.org/

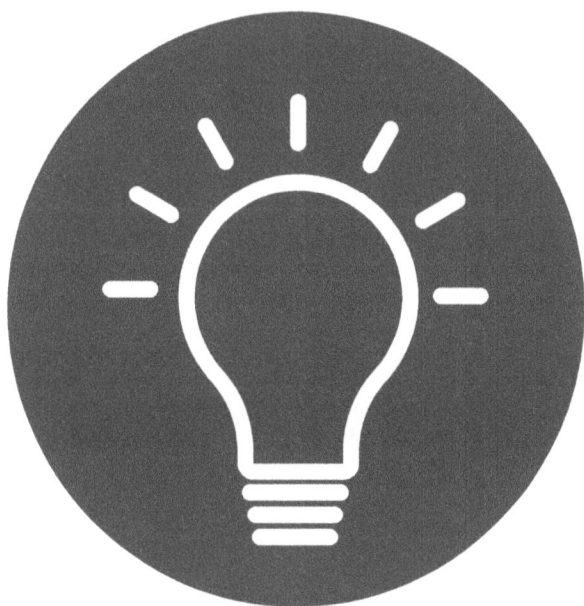

SUGGESTIONS

SLEEP

1. As you have previously read, sleep is extremely important. I would make sure that between the hours of 2-4 am you're asleep every night. At this time one should already be in a deep state of sleep so going to bed no later than 11:30 pm would be advisable.

FOOD

2. Ideally, one should not eat dinner no later than 6 pm. Why? Once food enters the stomach, it takes about 2 to 4 hours for it to move into the small intestine. From there, it takes about 4 to 6 hours for the food to pass through the small intestine and enter the large intestine (colon). If one eats late in the evening they're more than likely still processing their food at bed time, which disrupts the ability for many to enter into a deep state of sleep.

3. The heaviest meal of the day should not be Dinner.

4. Lunch time would be better for the heaviest meal as the body is in a more vibrant state and it will have more than enough time to digest before the evening sets in.

5. I would not follow the recommendations of the S.A.D. (Standard American Diet) as it puts too much emphasis on the consumption of grains.

CLEANING

6. I would suggest using dish washing soap or laundry detergent that does not have any added perfumes and dyes.

7. Clean clothes should have a neutral smell, and if a certain smell is needed there are natural alternatives then to bath your clothing and in-turn yourself with these toxic agents.

8. Adding a few drops of essential oil such as lavender or lemon to the rinse cycle can give the pleasant scent many long for in a more wholistic way.

PEACE

9. We consume in many ways such as by eating, reading, listening, and by what some called energy, feelings, a vibe.

10. Consuming (eating) what causes the body to fall out of balance causes illness. Instead we can choose to treat our body as a temple not to be defiled; we can mostly avoid the avenues of sickness.

11. Consuming (reading) foul reading material ingests these thoughts deeper into our minds as if speaking a sermon of these unholy scriptures within our temple. Again defiling it yet again. Instead be cautious and have discernment on what one reads as entertainment.

12. Consuming (listening) to the erratic thought forms, negativity and devious projections of those who we give our ear to may cause us to eventually act out in some way allowing us to be a vessel of these projections sometimes without even knowing. Instead be cautious on what you listen to, as all should uplift you during your days here within the realm, not tear your down.

13. Consuming (energetically) the negative energy (vibe) of others can lead to not noticing when something is amiss which could save our life, or long term exposure may lead to one taking on the ills in the form of physical or metaphysical misfortune. Let's start to work on trusting ourselves by becoming more sensitive to the mind, body, spirit connection by meditating. Just rhythmic breathing for at least 5 minutes daily. That's it!

CONTACT ME

In a time when many are suffering which I have found in many cases surrounds their consumption; I found it imperative to utilize my skills to help another. Which I hope has been helpful to you!

I've been studying, experiencing and teaching Alternative Health Modalities, S.T.E.M., Scientific Research, Horticulture, Metaphysics and more for decades; utilizing my gifts to bring waywardly spaces back into balance.

If needed I can be reached at:

www.TonyVortex.info

@VortexianSpin

@VortexianSpin

Here you will find links to:

- Consultations
- Events
- Herbs
- Books
- And more!

Love and Live!

Take Care,
Tony

www.ingramcontent.com/pod-product-compliance
Lightning Source LLC
Chambersburg PA
CBHW050844270326
41930CB00020B/3466